Putting Patients and Profits into Perspective

Michael E. Rindler

Pluribus Press, Chicago

Library of Congress Catalog Card Number:
86-63226

International Standard Book Number:
0-931028-80-9

Pluribus Press, Inc.
160 East Illinois Street
Chicago, Illinois 60611

91 90 89 88 87 5 4 3 2 1

Printed in the United States of America

Dedicated to Aloys Rindler Jr.,
my first and best leadership teacher

CONTENTS

FOREWORD

MICHAEL RINDLER'S BOOK is specifically addressed to the hospital field. I breathed a big sigh of relief when I read it. Here is why:

The issues in healthcare have changed dramatically over the last three decades:

- In the 1950s, healthcare was enjoying the era of discovering new clinical methods.
- In the 1960s, Hill-Burton funds, physician extenders, and regional medical programs were used to expand these discoveries away from academic university settings.
- In the 1970s, questions of cost were paramount and hospitals were fiercely regulated.
- In the 1980s, we are in the Alphabet Soup Era of PPOs, HMOs, IPAs, PROs, and what one observer calls OWAs (Other Weird Arrangements).

The reaction to these pressures by healthcare managers has been prospective payment panic and a cut-throat interpretation of competition. Without realizing it, hospital managers and industry leaders have gradually come to ignore the basics of successful healthcare. Instead, hospital leaders have been urged by their professional associations, by consultants, by financial advisors, and by attorneys to be combatants, rather than professionals . . . to be ***interested in patient care as a revenue-producing business, rather than being interested in the business of delivering good patient care.***

As Mr. Rindler accurately points out:

> "At most national meetings of hospital executives, there is much talk of reorganization, holding companies, vertical integration, diversification, and other strategies intended to imitate the corporate world. There appears to be little, if any, reflection on improving our effectiveness in providing patient care. This is not to say the corporate trend is bad for patients. On the contrary, consolidation of resources, economies of scale, etc., may enhance patient-care outcomes *if* these outcomes are kept firmly in mind *as* 'corporate restructuring' takes place."

Response to the pressures has often been without character.

Barbara Tuchman, in her book *March of Folly,* defines folly as the purposeful selection of strategies contrary to stated goals, when better, feasible alternatives are available. Recent examples of the march of folly in the healthcare field include:

- Interpreting marketing as hard-sell advertising. The backlash to unprofessional marketing is just beginning. One columnist writes that operations are not done for clinical indications anymore, but have become "products peddled in the new American marketplace."
- Are hospitals solving the problem of funding indigent care? Yes. By being sure this hospital is a dumper, not a dumpee.

- In one hospital, a memo from a concerned cardiologist points out that obtaining the patient's chest x-ray as an outpatient endangers possible heart attack patients, and that it is being done not for clinical indications, but to maximize hospital reimbursement.

- Management has been superficial. "Our awnings are over the front door and our guest relations program is popular and our candlelight dinner is ready . . . We're a little short of nurses, so get your own wheelchair."

- The vice presidents of marketing and planning are in the carpeted wing of the hospital . . . quality assurance is in the basement by the boiler room, with no secretary.

Michael Rindler makes us recognize these faults. He makes us face ourselves, he brings us up short, and he forces us to reconsider our whole approach to hospital management. His book accurately foresees (without saying so) the hospital of 1995:

- Community health care services, of all types—not 95 percent of dollars and efforts committed to horizontal, in-bed patient care.

- A board of half business people and half professional people.

- Responsiveness to community needs and to lay advisory councils.

- A medical staff that is a true partner, not just a dotted line on an organizational chart to be worked around in Machiavellian fashion.

In this environment, the effective Chief Executive Officer

must be a well rounded leader, not a narrowly focused specialist who never developed a broad outlook.

Michael Rindler's book not only helps us recognize how far off track we have been, but tells us *how* to get back *on* track! This book is required reading for anyone who presumes to have the knowledge and skills to lead a hospital successfully during the next five to ten years . . . including next year . . . including tomorrow.

RICHARD E. THOMPSON, M.D.
President
Thompson, Mohr & Associates, Inc.

INTRODUCTION

Positive Patient Outcomes

THIS IS AN EXCITING time to be a hospital leader. The pace of technological change is accelerating. Financial pressures are sweeping weak hospitals away. For the first time, hospitals are competing for customers. Other businesses have done this for centuries. Only the best and most capable individuals will lead hospitals successfully into the future.

This book is about getting back to the basics. It is about leading, rather than merely managing a hospital. It is about rolling up our sleeves and getting in touch with our customers, hospital patients. This book is written from the point of view of a hospital chief executive officer for other chief executive officers and their senior management staff. Since the titles for senior managers vary considerably, we will use the term "senior management" to apply to vice presidents, assistant administrators, administrative directors, chief financial officers, and so on. These are our hospital leaders. They will inevitably take their hospitals to new levels of success or preside over their sad decline.

Patients expect our hospital leaders to produce positive outcomes on their behalf. Whether they are severely ill in an intensive care unit or undergoing a routine outpatient exam, patients need and expect to have services delivered with efficiency, quality, and economy. Patients care little about the "delivery system" or the process by which services are rendered. Hospital leaders are not paying enough attention to basic patient outcomes. Many are becoming too focused on the processes and systems which claim to produce positive outcomes on the patient's behalf.

A little perspective

Military history contains many references to the disadvantages of process orientation versus outcome orientation. Perhaps the most familiar is our own War of Independence. The British army was the epitome of process warfare. British soldiers marched, fought, and died in brightly colored red uniforms, in precise columns, using tactics based on rules and tradition. The colonists, on the other hand, cared little about traditional warfare. To them, the outcome of winning independence was of utmost importance. Little attention was paid to uniforms or the rules and traditions of warfare. The colonists concentrated on winning battles in whatever way they could. It was their exclusive focus on the outcome of winning which enabled them to defeat what was then the most powerful army on earth.

The essence of leadership in hospitals is to produce positive outcomes for patients. Hospitals are in business to help sick people get better when cure or improvement is within the scope of our skills and technology, and to relieve the suffering of and provide a humane, dignified and sensitive environment for, those beyond hope and medical capabilities. A hospital outcome in its best and purest form is a patient who recovers from an illness or surgery. Each hospital department has a number of specific and measurable patient outcomes. These include items such as hot and attractively served food, a clean and pleasant environment, accurate laboratory studies, clinically significant x-ray exams performed on a timely basis, rehabilitation treatments that actually accomplish intended goals, delivery of nursing treatments and medication in accordance with physician orders, and others.

Patients have no interest in process

Understandably, patients do not care about process; they care about outcomes. Patients do not appreciate the elegance of a quality control system in a hospital kitchen which assures excellent meals and superbly controlled temperatures on the assembly line, but still results in cold food at the bedside. Patients worry as they watch the IV fluid level drop to a point that they fear is dangerously low. Patients are justifiably angry when kept NPO (without food and water) for hours after an appointed time for a diagnostic test only to be told that it has been cancelled due to equipment failure. How fast the business office can produce an itemized statement is of far less concern to the patient than how fast a nurse or aide can present them with a bed pan in their time of need. It is toward these kinds of patient outcomes that hospital leaders need, increasingly, to direct their attention.

Admittedly, it is easier to emphasize style and process. When one focuses on process, one can always tinker under the guise of "refining." Since there are no perfect systems, there is no end to the tinkering. How many times have chief executive officers heard the plea that if we just had one more month or ten thousand more dollars, we could finally solve the "linen problem" or finally achieve the definitive "patient classification system"? In the endless search to improve systems and the process by which outcomes are produced, we often lose sight of the product which those systems are supposed to produce.

When process becomes more important than outcomes

Hospitals are full of process orientation examples. One is the emphasis on staff functions, such as planning, marketing, and management information systems. It is not unusual to find vice presidential level personnel in one or all of these positions even in small hospitals. Many hospital leaders fail to ask the key question: "What are these staff functions doing for our patients?" Good leadership and focus on positive patient outcomes is still one of the most effective public relations and marketing strategies for any hospital. Staff functions are powerful tools, but they should not become substitutes for good line management and producing satisfied customers.

A second example is the "corporate" trend. At most national meetings of hospital executives there is much talk of reorganization, holding companies, vertical integration, diversification and other strategies intended to imitate the successful corporate sector. There appears to be little, if any, reflection on improving patient care. It is as if our primary service, patient care, is only an ancillary concern. This is not to say that the corporate trend is bad for patients. On the contrary, consolidation of resources, economies of scale, and so on may enhance patient care outcomes if these outcomes are kept firmly in mind during and after the "corporate restructuring."

Increasing dependence on consultants is a third example. As we depend more on complex systems, we are depending more on outside consultation. One indication of growth in the number of consultants is membership in the American Association of Healthcare Consultants. In 1972 there were approximately 25 member firms and 100 individuals; by 1986, the number had grown to 98 firms and 233 individuals.[1] This does not include the thousands of consultants who do not belong to the prestigious AAHC. Although most dollars spent on consulting services are justified, a good portion of the consultation fees paid by hospitals are for reports and services which will never produce a single positive outcome for patients.

What has happened to management basics?

Process orientation is further stimulated by the decreasing emphasis on the basics of management by hospital administrative staffs. Senior hospital management are recruited primarily from MHA and MBA programs. The overwhelming focus of these programs is analytical and technical. Little in the academic sojourn prepares graduates for the real world of hospital leadership.

The real world entails dealing with such practical situations as dietary workers upset by their low status; astronomical lab costs resulting from medical resident ordering patterns; the identity crisis of registered nurses and the frustration and anger that it evokes; dealing with an alcoholic department manager or head nurse. This type of human relations problem solving is not addressed in today's master's degree programs. Consequently, new administrative staff members are ill-prepared for real world management issues.

Even senior administrative staff members often know little about the patient care outcomes produced by the departments for which they are responsible. Perhaps they have confused being a boss with being a leader. An essential element of their leadership is the ability to keep middle managers focused on producing desired outcomes. Do hospital leaders have sustained ability and sustained dedication to their product, patient care? Unfortunately, many do not.

The ability to identify positive patient outcomes and keep middle managers and employees focused on producing them is essential. It is far more important than the organizational structure, the elegance of financial control systems, or the size of the planning department. The focus on process in our institutions is likely to produce several negative by-products. First, and most importantly, such a focus may de-emphasize patient care outcomes.

If hospital leaders let their middle managers measure success in terms of growing budgets, acquiring sophisticated equipment and adding more personnel, the tendency will be to increase costs with no consideration as to what costs contribute to patient care. Regrettably, staff departments such as planning, marketing, and information systems are taking an increasingly larger role in our institutions. But are they contributing to positive patient outcomes? Their growth, in part, is because they have become strong advocates of their own self interest.

Thomas J. Peters and Robert H. Waterman Jr.'s study of America's best run corporations shows that, above all, excellent companies were brilliant on the basics. Tools didn't substitute for thinking. Intellect didn't overcome wisdom. Analysis didn't impede action. Rather, these companies worked hard to keep things simple in a complex world. They persisted. They insisted on top quality. They focused on their customers. They listened to employees and treated them like adults. IBM, Hewlett-Packard, Delta Airlines, Procter & Gamble, among others, have enjoyed sustained success by paying attention to the basics and to customer outcomes, not by focusing on process.[2] The lessons we learn from these successful corporations should be applied to the leading of hospitals.

Renewed emphasis on patients

We need to re-emphasize, at all levels of our organizations, the basic fact that hospitals exist to serve patient needs. Hospital leaders need to remind themselves constantly that one of their principle responsibilities is to ensure that patient care is delivered in the most effective way possible. They need to capitalize on the fact that administrative staffs and department managers take their cues from CEOs and senior management. If leaders talk about and focus on process, so will their staffs. If, on the other hand, leaders constantly focus on patient outcomes, management staffs will devote their energies and attention to patient outcomes. That is leading by example.

Second, hospital leaders should get closer to their customers, patients. Carrying out our ''executive duties'' includes listening to patients' suggestions and hearing their perceptions about the care received in our institutions. Listening proves we cannot assume because a system or process is in place that the intended positive patient outcomes will automatically follow. We should make sure the outcome is produced, reviewing with our managers the obstacles to achievement as we check back periodically to see that delivery is sustained.

Third, we should begin to evaluate institutional changes more carefully, such as equipment purchases, staff additions, and system changes, in terms of what they will do for patients in addition to what they will do for an individual department or physician. When management evaluations begin to be based on contributions to patient care objectives, we should begin to see a constructive change in attitude and better use of scarce financial resources. It will also put those analytical skills acquired in graduate school to far better use than designing the "ultimate" system.

Hospital CEOs should keep in mind that advanced education does not necessarily prepare competent line managers in a hospital setting. When new graduates assume responsibility for departments, they should learn those departments thoroughly, especially the outcomes that department produces for patients. Leaders need to keep department managers focused on patient outcomes through the questions that they ask daily and in the evaluations performed on the department managers' effectiveness. They should be certain that department managers do not become so focused on process that it becomes an end it itself.

Hospital leaders should focus their management staffs on improving outcomes for their patients and working with them to think across departmental lines. The outcome of this emphasis may ensure that an NPO patient has a meal when returning from radiology, or that a patient's family gets timely information when a loved one emerges from surgery. All hospital leaders from junior members to the CEO should appreciate the inherent complexity of producing outcomes which matter to patients. That "team" focus then needs to be instilled at all levels of the organization so that everyone is working for the patient's benefit rather than solely for a narrowly-focused department or personal interest.

Cultivating a caring attitude

Where does an increased emphasis on outcomes lead? It may lead to tackling the really difficult issues, like cultivating a positive and caring attitude in all employees. Perhaps it will lead to radiologists reducing patient waiting time and overcharges resulting from the ordering of routine chest and skull x-rays for screening purposes. Utilization studies have shown these studies make little contribution to patient diagnosis and treatment. Or maybe it will lead to pathologists teaching their fellow physicians that they do not need to order routine urine and hematology studies with every admission. Studies have shown these also to be of minimal value. Increased emphasis on outcomes will clarify issues that really make a difference in our patients' care and what they pay for it.

Insight worth more to patients than process

Management authors Robert H. Hays and William J. Abernathy commented, "We believe that during the past two decades, American managers have increasingly relied on principles which prize analytical detachment and methodological elegance over insight. . . based on experience."[3] This statement is as germane to hospital leadership as it is to business. Hospital executives, in their attempt to build better corporate structures, more advanced systems and more medical technology, should not forget that the basic mission of hospitals is to care for sick people.

What can we call a leadership approach which emphasizes patient outcomes and de-emphasizes process? Many labels were considered, but most of the creative ones seem to have already been claimed. ''Simple-minded management'' describes the basic thrust but may be construed as a reference to the intellect of those who practice it. Perhaps we should simply call it ''Back to the Patients.''

PART ONE

LEADERSHIP VALUES

CHAPTER ONE

Leadership Job One: Corporate Values

WALT DISNEY knew about the importance of corporate values. He may be best remembered by the general public for his creative film making genius, Mickey Mouse, and Disney Land; but he assured his place in business history by creating an organization which is still successfully driven by basic principles of customer service and economic value. Even today, no one goes to work at Disney World without first attending ''school'' to learn the corporate values of the Disney Organization. Disney instills corporate values in its people as well if not better than any company in the U.S. today. Hospital leaders can learn something special from Disney—the necessity of having and teaching corporate values to their staffs.

It is the job of hospital leaders, CEOs and senior management to define clearly the values of their organizations. Those values should flow from a board developed mission statement which defines the overall expectations for the organization. The mission statement should not be one of those three page motherhood and apple pie documents which is filed on a shelf and never sees the light of day. A mission statement should be concise and accurately reflect the board's goals for the organization.

Is there any doubt about what the mission statement says about quality for the Rolls Royce Corporation? Is there any doubt that IBM's mission is to be the best in service, or that Hewlett-Packard's is to be the best in technological innovation? Hospital missions may range from the "friendly" mission of the community hospital to the "teaching" and "research" missions of university medical centers. Regardless of a hospital's mission, a set of central corporate values is necessary for the mission to be fulfilled, day in and day out by its employees.

The CEO and senior management's job is to establish and articulate those values. Five corporate values used by a Wisconsin community hospital present an excellent example of how to create and instill values in a hospital work force. The five values are: honesty and integrity; pride and quality; hard work; communication; and customer service. These five values would serve any hospital well, regardless of its mission.

Honesty and integrity

Hospital leaders should expect their employees to deal with their organization with honesty and integrity. After all, that is what employees expect of their leaders. But how often do hospital leaders articulate honesty as an expectation for their employees? Some may put it in their employee handbook along with a lot of other "boiler plate." But taking an extra step and looking employees in the eye and telling them personally that their leaders expect them to deal with their organization honestly is what is really needed.

Honesty means not calling in sick once a month simply because an employee thinks a hospital owes him a sick day. Sick time abuse is probably the single greatest example of lack of employee honesty in hospitals. Why is that?

It's because hospital leaders have not done a good enough job explaining the difference between an entitlement benefit like vacation and a protective benefit like sick time.

Hospitals are full of examples of honesty and integrity problems. They lose supplies and equipment every day. Why? Because people steal and waste them. Although hospitals terminate an occasional employee when they are fortunate enough to catch them, many times they simply miss the thefts and waste. There would be a lot less stealing and wasting in hospitals if their leaders made a point of telling employees that they expected them to treat their hospitals like their own household. They should explain the facts of life to employees about how dollars lost from theft and waste come out of everyone's pocket and make unavailable new employee benefits and improvements in patient services.

Honesty and integrity are also related to patient confidentiality. It is a shame some hospitals do not pay more attention to confidentiality. Patients entrust themselves to hospitals for their care, and do not expect to have their various ailments and diseases talked about in the staff cafeteria or over drinks in the local bar. But that can and does happen in hospitals every day. Leaders should look their staff in the eye and tell them they expect honesty and integrity. They should remind their staff frequently about this, and stress that there are no exceptions. It takes a certain amount of courage and the ability to set a positive example to carry this off effectively. Hospital leaders must be up to the task.

Pride and quality

You can really tell the difference between a hospital whose employees are focused on pride and quality and one that is not. You can even tell a difference from department to department in the same hospital just by making some quick observations. Consider the meal that was just delivered to the patient bedside. Is it hot, does it taste good, does it look good? If so, it is the mark of pride and quality in a dietary department and its staff. Are the floors clean? Do the bathrooms sparkle? If so, those are the marks of pride and quality in a housekeeping department, not the size of their policy and procedure manual.

Hospital leaders should expect that each and every employee take pride in their individual job and that they take pride in producing a quality product or service for their individual departments. An employee who has no pride is an unhappy employee and an attitude problem waiting to happen. My advice for hospital leaders when they discover employees who have bad attitudes and little pride is to encourage them to go to work for one of your competitors. I do not mean to sound facetious. On the contrary, to find a poor attitude employee and not do anything about it is a symptom of poor leadership. If you cannot put pride and quality into an employee, get a new employee who has or can learn those attributes.

Pride is demonstrated in a number of ways, from the appearance of the employee and the department in which he or she works to the output or service for which he or she is responsible. It is the hospital leadership's job to be sure that every employee knows that they are expected to produce at that level. Employees should further understand that if they are incapable of producing at that level then their continued presence will not be required.

Hard work

The work ethic of employees varies from hospital to hospital—some cynics might even say from day to day in the same hospital. It is the hospital leadership's job to establish the work ethic for their organization. Hard work by all employees at all times should be a corporate value in all hospitals. Some might snicker at the notion of articulating a hard day's work as a corporate value. "Isn't it self evident?" they would say. Hardly. The work ethic in hospitals varies from excellent to dismal, with a much heavier leaning towards the dismal side. It is the CEOs and senior management's job to let their employees know they expect them to work hard, to work smart, and to work cooperatively with their fellow employees, managers, and physicians.

What does this mean on a day-to-day basis? It means not taking extended lunch hours and coffee breaks. It means coming to work on time, and not leaving early. It means giving their full attention to the job every minute they are at work. It means not studying for a school exam on the evening shift, or doing a macramé plant hanger on an IV stand on the night shift. It means giving full attention to the job. When there are activity lulls, it means going out and looking for other work to do.

We do not have enough of the "old-fashioned" work ethic in hospitals today. It is part of the reason why some hospitals are in such dire financial straits, and even going bankrupt. If every hospital leader took pains to let their employees know that they expected them to work hard every day, there would be some amazing increases in productivity. The best corporate leaders do not seem to have much trouble demanding hard work from their employees in industry, and we should not have much trouble doing so either.

Communication

Communication is a corporate value of the highest importance. Hospital leaders must be both communicators and listeners. They must also articulate the need for employees to communicate and listen as well. Communication can be divided into two major components: communication with customers and communication with the organization. We will discuss first communication with the customer.

A good place to start in talking about customer communication is how hospital employees address patients. Do they call them "sweetie pie," "honey," "dearie"? Many nurses do. Perhaps they do it as a sign of affection, but most patients do not like to be called "sweetie pie." They would much rather be called by their real name. Staff should not even presume to use a patient or family member's first name unless they are asked to do so. Given the choice, an elderly gentleman would probably prefer to be called "Mr. Wood" instead of "dearie." Using a customer's name is one small way of communicating that we respect his or her dignity. It is an opportunity which should not be lost.

Another customer communication issue is door knocking. When staff members enter a patient room they should knock on the door, even if the door is open. They should introduce themselves by name. And they should take pains to say hello to the patient in the other bed if it is an occupied semi-private room. Even if hospital staffs have no duties to perform with the other patient, they should at least say hello and acknowledge their presence.

Staffs should be able to communicate appropriately with customers with reference to service delays. We all know that it is impossible to deliver instantaneously every pain medication or bed pan. However, the staff may exercise various options in communicating the reasons for delay. Those options range from telling the patient the hospital is "understaffed," to a more appropriate response that the service will be delivered in ten minutes because an emergency situation has to be attended to first. The way that our staff communicates service delays makes a tremendous difference in the attitudes our customers develop about the hospital.

Our staffs should be instructed to greet and say hello to everyone they have contact with in the hospital. This means instructing the staff to say hello to passing visitors, employees, and patients in the corridors. It takes a little getting used to, but incorporating this behavior into the hospital's value system will create an overall environment which is very customer friendly. If implemented effectively, hospitals might even have employees saying hello to visitors in the elevator, instead of staring at the ceiling or down at the floor or every other place but where the customers are.

Communication within the organization is also very important. Many of the registered nurse union organizing campaigns taking place around the country today have nothing to do with wages, hours, or working conditions. They have everything to do, however, with communication and input into the patient care process. There have been many unenlightened organizations who have lost elections on the simple issue of communication.

To be effective, communication means creating an avenue for both ideas and concerns of staff members to flow freely upward and downward. It is the CEO and senior management's obligation to let it be known that they expect their staff to communicate both upward and downward. They should make it known that they expect employees to communicate all the way to the top if not satisfied through the normal communication channels. They should, in fact, implement both formal and informal communication channels to make certain that the staff members are both communicating and listening effectively. Staff members should feel free to write a memo to the CEO or stop him or her in the corridor without fear.

A hospital leader's effectiveness in articulating the communication value is important for the successful integration of all other values. It is the leader's obligation to set a good example. How can an uncommunicative CEO expect a nurses' aide to communicate and listen at the bedside if his or her communication is not effective? How can they instill their vision of the organization's future unless the CEO can articulate it in a way everyone can understand? It is the hospital leadership's job to create opportunities to communicate constantly. It is also their job to instill in employees the understanding that communication is expected, not optional.

Customer service

It has been said many times that customers could get better and friendlier service at any Sears store than they could in most hospitals. Why is that so? It is because Sears figured out a long time ago that a dissatisfied customer could go to J.C. Penney's, Montgomery Ward, or some other competitor. Until recently, those of us in the hospital business had not figured that out. Hospital leaders should ensure that each employee understands that patients and their family are the customers. They should also understand that going the extra mile for customers is expected behavior rather than a rare event.

Industry is full of wonderful examples of going the extra mile for customers. Some particularly interesting ones are from American Express. Their stories are almost unbelievable. For example, customer service people in the Florida Operations Center found a way to get money and a steamship booking to a woman stranded in a hotel in war torn Beruit. Travel agents in Columbus, Georgia, bailed a French journalist out of jail. A travel counselor in New York drove through a blizzard to deliver food and blankets to travelers stranded at Kennedy Airport. A travel agent in Boston managed to re-unite a non-English speaking Japanese mother, stranded in Boston because of a diverted flight, with her daughter in Philadelphia. As touching as these stories are for their purely human interest, they are also intriguing examples of living corporate legends that illustrate that an organization does value customer service.[4]

Hospital leaders must instill in their staff a reverence for their customers. Remember, customers are not only our patients, but our patients' families, their friends and neighbors, who may visit or inquire about them. I wonder how many times a family member has been told that "I don't know the answer about how your mother is because I am not working on that team tonight." On the other hand, many employees in our hospitals today have gotten the message to the extent that they would go to any lengths to get answers about a patient's condition to a distraught family member.

I once heard of a nurse who comforted a new mother at 2 a.m. by bringing her newborn to the bedside after the mother thought she heard her infant crying. Even though the nurse knew it was physically impossible for the infant to be heard in the mother's room, even if it was crying, she knew the best way to reassure the mother was to bring her sleeping infant to her.

Hospital leaders must instill in their staffs the ability to be flexible so that they can go the extra mile. Staffs should not be so tied to "policy" that they do not let a visitor stay an extra few minutes in the Intensive Care Unit with a dying family member. On the contrary, if this customer service value has been instilled appropriately, staff members will go out of their way to look for opportunities to demonstrate flexibility with the customers.

Now that the competitive revolution has reached our industry we need to focus more clearly on our customers and customer service. We need to make up for lost time and be sure that all of our employees have gotten the customer service message. It's the job of hospital leaders to be sure that they do.

Internalizing corporate values

How does a hospital leader, particularly the CEO, communicate corporate values to his many employees? As a start he does it by participating in new employee orientations. No matter how large the hospital, the CEO should take enough time to be first on the agenda at all new employee orientations. In that orientation, he should explain exactly what the hospital corporate values are and what they mean to individual employees. He should also explain what he expects from them and what they can expect of their organization in return. He should let them know that he expects them to: be honest; take pride in the quality of their work; work hard; communicate effectively; and above all practice the art of customer service.

The CEO and his senior management should then reinforce those values at periodic formal employee meetings. They should give employees examples of what they are talking about and how it applies in their particular departments. They should explain how the achievement of those values is fulfilling the hospital's mission to the community. They should give employees the corporate values statement in writing as well, and they should ask enough questions periodically to assure themselves that employees understand and have internalized those values.

Repetition never hurts when it comes to corporate values. Figure I illustrates the approach and responsibilities for achieving employee internalization of a hospital's corporate values.

Teaching corporate values to the entire staff may sound like a tall order to some hospital leaders. If intimidated, I suggest they study Jan Carlson's approach to turning around SAS Airlines in the early 1980s. Carlson personally preached the value of enhanced service, creativity, and finding a better way to 20,000 SAS employees. His monumental effort helped lead SAS out of period of lackluster performance to become one of the most successful and profitable airlines in aviation history.

FIGURE 1

CORPORATE VALUES

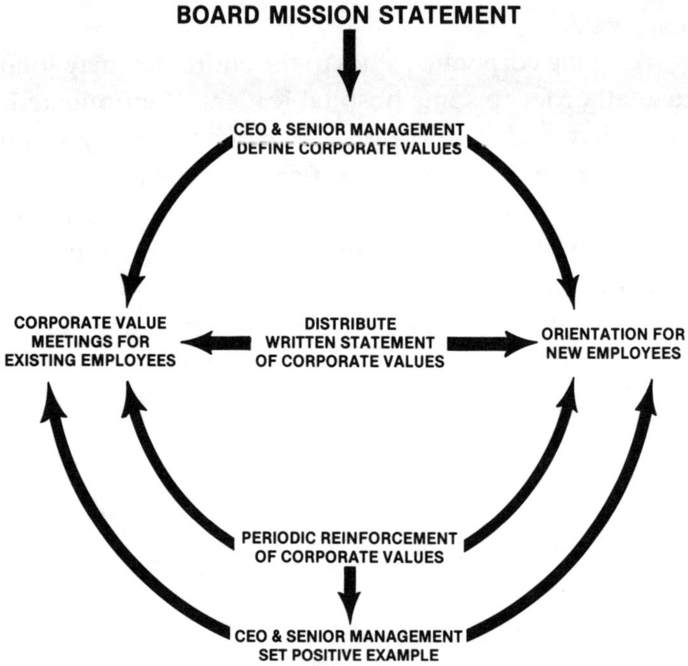

CHAPTER TWO

The Leadership Example: They Always Notice

HOSPITAL EMPLOYEES take their cue from their leaders. Employees, volunteers, and even physicians pick up subtle and sometimes not so subtle signals transmitted by CEOs and senior management. Competence, commitment, physical appearance, mood, and even tone of voice can influence and quickly affect the morale of hundreds of individuals associated with the hospital.

Hospital leaders are observed and scrutinized like no other member of the organization. Where they park their car, the color and quality of their clothes, the expression on their faces, and the level of their competence are the subject of discussion daily. This assumes of course that they venture out of their offices enough to be noticed. The CEO and senior management set the values for their organization. They should also set the standard for following those values.

Any sign of inconsistency in living the organization's values by the CEO or by the senior management is instantly transmitted throughout the organization through its grapevine. Hypocritical leaders are soon discovered in a hospital setting. Hospital leaders may use their organization's grapevine to strengthen corporate values through example. On the other hand, it may be their downfall if they do not practice what they preach.

How do CEOs and senior management "practice what they preach"? By living the corporate values that they establish for their organization. A few examples, using the corporate values discussed in Chapter 1, illustrate how leaders can live their hospital's corporate values.

Pride and quality

Hospital leaders set the tone with reference to pride in their organization and quality of work. Do the leaders have pride in their personal appearance, the appearance of their work space, and the appearance of their organization? If they do, it will be clearly evident. If they do not, it will be just as evident.

Appearance and the symbols of pride are definitely important for all hospital leaders. Employees and customers know a faker when they see one. How can a hospital leader market wellness programs if he is forty pounds overweight and a two pack a day smoker? Obviously he cannot. How can an assistant administrator expect the housekeeping department to take pride in cleaning patient rooms if his own office looks like a tornado has recently struck? There are countless ways leaders can use visible symbols of pride and quality to their great advantage. These visible symbols can set a very high standard of excellence for the rest of the organization.

Bill Marriott, President of the Marriott Hotel Corporation, demonstrates his commitment to pride and quality by frequently walking unannounced into storerooms in his hotels. He looks for the cleanliness of stored dinner plates, among other things.[5] His passion for quality and attention to detail is legendary, partly because he makes those surprise inspections to check on dinner plates.

The personal quality of a leader's work is also another opportunity for setting positive examples. Producing a slipshod report or accepting poor quality work from a subordinate becomes the organizational standard if its leaders allow it. On the other hand, striving for excellence and constantly stimulating the organization to higher levels of performance sets a positive example that quickly is replicated throughout the organization. Leaders hold in their power the ability to bring their organizations to record high levels of performance, or to drag them down into mediocrity. The pride which they take in their own work and the quality of their personal work performance is the key factor in deciding which direction their organization will move.

The work ethic

Hospital leaders are the principle standard setters with reference to work ethic. Their starting hours in the morning and quitting times in the evening are closely observed. The time leaders spend at lunch is a source of afternoon gossip if it is even thirty seconds past the organization's alotted time. Off hours presence in the hospital is instantly noticed and communicated throughout the hospital. If a leader periodically does some of his work or goes on rounds in the evening, night, or weekend hours he can be assured that his presence will be instantly known throughout the hospital.

I am reminded of how fast word can travel when recalling an incident many years ago when making a tour of my hospital at 2 a.m. After walking through a nursing unit for a few minutes, I found no one in sight. Since the telephone was persistently ringing at the nursing station, I answered it. A hushed voice said, without introduction, "Watch out, the boss is in the building again." The mystery of how word travelled so quickly during my off hours visit was solved. The switchboard had acted with lightning speed to report to each nursing unit and department that "the boss" was making rounds.

The way hospital leaders use their working time is also a subject of much comment among their staff. If they are productive and use their time well it sets a positive example for doing likewise throughout the hospital. If, on the other hand, they enjoy extended socializing to the detriment of their other responsibilities, that is also duly imprinted in the minds of the staff. The individuals who notice a leader's work ethic most are the hospital's middle management staff.

The CEO's interaction with his subordinates and associates is the subject of much discussion among those subordinates. Any hint of hypocritical behavior quickly becomes a matter of detrimental conversation. Whether the CEO and senior managers realize it or not, their credibility can be significantly compromised if they do not practice what they preach.

The trust and consideration shown for subordinates is a key factor in having those subordinates internalize the organization's corporate values. A CEO who espouses trust and common courtesy but does not practice it himself is appropriately labeled a hypocrite. A leader who keeps his subordinates waiting, who frequently cancels appointments, and who continues working and accepting phone calls while meeting with those subordinates, should not be at all surprised to learn that those subordinates interact with their employees in the same discourteous way.

Many hospital leaders are tremendously hard workers. They should realize, however, that merely working hard is not enough. They must work hard in a fashion that provides a positive leadership example for their subordinates and for the entire hospital staff. By being conscious of the example they are setting for others, they will maximize their role as the work ethic standard setter for the rest of the organization.

Communicating and listening

It is easy to talk, but not so easy to listen. Hospital leaders must be excellent role models for their managers and employees when it comes to communication. Mainly, this means being accessible and placing a high value on personal communication.

Hospital leaders must be the visible practitioners of effective communication. They should always remember to knock before entering a patient's room, address patients by their last name, and always ensure that patient and family concerns are promptly addressed. There are some excellent examples of CEOs and senior management using symbols to illustrate their commitment to communication. One Midwest CEO goes as far as placing his personal office telephone number in the hospital's newspaper advertisements. He further invites anyone reading the newspaper to call him directly if they have a concern about the hospital's performance, or an idea to improve it. The CEO has learned that only a few people take the time and effort to call him; however, those who do either have something very positive or very negative to say. Those calls give the CEO and senior management opportunities to set a good follow up example for the rest of their organization.

The CEO tells the story of receiving a call from a disgruntled patient several days after one of the ads with his phone number appeared in the local newspaper. The patient described her situation as follows:

> "I read your newspaper ad and decided to call you even though I know it will not do any good. I had my first baby in your hospital four years ago and I have been mad ever since. I was keeping a momento book for my baby, and wanted to place his nursery wristband in the book. But your nurses lost it. So what are you going to do about my problem?"

Without batting an eye, the CEO had the nursery staff prepare a new wristband with the infant's patient information as it appeared at birth. That evening, on his way home, the CEO dropped it off at the caller's home. Within days, the surprised mother spread the story throughout the whole neighborhood that the hospital CEO was a man of his word. The story also circulated quickly throughout the hospital and created an excellent example of the CEO's commitment to be accessible and resolve problems when once surfaced. Admittedly, most problems are much more difficult to resolve, but the symbolic value of the hospital's leadership listening and then taking action puts the organization in the correct frame of mind for responding to the more difficult situations which inevitably surface.

Leaders should also set the example when communicating within the organization. They do this best by communicating personally, rather than delegating. Effective leaders do not depend on newsletters to communicate with their employees; they do it personally. For example, attending new employee orientations give leaders the opportunity to establish from the very beginning that communication is an important value. There is just no substitute for leaders themselves setting a positive example for the entire staff by communicating personally.

Honesty and integrity

The CEO and senior management must set the example for the hospital staff when it comes to honesty and integrity. It is well known that a number of hospital leaders and senior managers have lost their jobs through dishonesty such as misusing hospital funds. Although it may take awhile, anyone in a high position who is dishonest will ultimately be discovered and ultimately discharged. Hospital leaders must also set the tone for honesty and integrity by always being forthright in their communications with employees, physicians, and their board. Being evasive or selectively admitting "bad news" has been the downfall of many hospital leaders.

The use of hospital funds and property for personal gain sets an extremely poor example. There is no need to dwell on the "horror stories" which recount hospital CEOs using their engineering staffs to remodel their personal kitchen or repave their driveway. If hospital leaders are misusing their positions in that way, employees will know about it and laugh behind their backs if they try to espouse honesty and integrity as a corporate value.

The hospital CEO and senior management have a tremendous amount of trust placed in them. The trust begins with their board and ends with their employees and community. They should always perform their responsibilities in a manner that sets the highest possible example for the rest of their organization.

Patients as customers

Hospital leaders should set the example for treating patients as customers. They can do this first and foremost by frequently talking with patients, a sometimes unheard-of concept for today's busy hospital executives. Talking with and listening to the customers in their rooms, in the x-ray department, in the emergency room waiting area, is behavior that gets observed by other employees and members of the management staff.

There are many opportunities to do this, from chatting with families in the elevator to spending a few minutes with them in the lobby as patients are discharged. Senior management must also set positive examples. Having the vice president of nursing spend a few minutes in the emergency room waiting area several times a week with families quickly lets the nursing staff know how interested that leader is in good service.

A hospital in Minneapolis has leadership who really practice the approach of getting close to the customer. At 5:30 a.m. each weekday senior executives start work by talking with patients who are arriving for day surgery procedures. Early each morning these leaders get a dose of patient care reality direct from their customers. They set a tremendous example for their hospital staff and for the hospital industry.

Hospital leaders cannot say they are "patient oriented" and then never speak to patients. You would be surprised at how many leaders do just that. If hospital leaders passed a few dietary trays or answered a few requests for bed pans now and then they would find their staff responding in an extremely positive way. Frequent contact with patients and their families by hospital leaders is a tremendous way to set the example. We can take a "customer service" lesson from John Scully, Chairman of the Apple Computer Corporation. He regularly takes a turn at Apple's toll-free customer service number answering questions and following up product complaints.[6] If he can do it, so can we.

The power of leadership

What two things do these five men have in common: William Watson Jr.,; Walt Disney; Harold Geneen; Alfred P. Sloan; and Arnold S. Anderson, M.D.? Each man achieved legendary status in leading their respective organizations. They were strong leaders whose personal and corporate values were deeply imprinted on their staffs.

Each man also retired after more than two decades of successful leadership. They were not "flashes in the pan," but genuine leadership success stories who stood the test of time. Personally setting the leadership example for their organizations and practicing corporate values were important factors in their success.

The first four names are familiar ones. They led IBM, Disney Productions, ITT, and General Motors respectively. Dr. Anderson is not a household name, but his achievements as a legendary leader are just as great. Dr. Anderson was the founder and driving force behind the Minneapolis Children's Medical Center. Upon his retirement in January 1986, here are just a few of the hundreds of comments made about him as published in the Medical Center's "Children's Hour" magazine in its Winter 1986 edition:

> "He was our leader, our mentor, and our inspiration."
>
> "Dr. Anderson is our walking mission statement. He provides stability, rationality, enthusiasm, coaching, cheerleading, guidance, cajoling, and above all teaching in all of the above."

> "Arne is one of those rare breeds of people who possess an ability to mix idealism with realism and take an organization into uncharted waters."

> "Arne's most significant contribution has been his unwaving commitment to the mission statement and his dedication to implementing it through his own example. . . ."

Leading by example. If leaders aspire to greatness, their organizations will follow as Dr. Anderson's did. What greater compliment can an organization bestow on its leader than saying he is their "walking mission statement"?

CHAPTER THREE

Communication: Make It Personal

MANY HOSPITALS have lost the art of being personal. So have some hospital leaders. They rely on staffs and surrogate systems far too often to communicate with customers, physicians, employees, and sometimes even the community. Hospital leaders need to devote a major portion of their time communicating. There is no substitute for doing it personally, not even elegant newsletters or videotaped "personal" messages.

Communicating with patients

Hospital leaders must make the time to talk with their customers. Who are they? They are, of course, the inpatients who entrust themselves to our care. But our customers are also sitting in our emergency room waiting rooms, waiting for a loved one or friend. They are in our x-ray rooms, having blood drawn in our laboratories, and rebuilding muscle strength in our physical therapy departments.

Hospital leaders must ensure that customers have every opportunity to express concerns. An unusually conclusive set of studies of consumer complaint behavior was carried out during the Carter Administration by a Washington, D.C.

company called Technical Assistance Research Programs, Inc. (TARP). The TARP study demonstrated that the average business never hears from 96 percent of its unhappy customers. It further pointed out that for every complaint received, there are an average of 26 other customers with problems. Finally, the study concluded that the average dissatisfied customer tells ten people about their negative experience.[7] Hospitals are not immune from this phenomenon and must act with creativity to receive and follow up on negative customer experiences.

Hospital leaders can learn a great deal by setting aside a few minutes regularly to talk with customers directly. This is commonly known as "rounds." Some of the more recently articulate writers on management call it "management by wandering around." Whatever it is called, it is every bit as important for hospital leaders to talk to their customers as it is for the chairman of an airline to ride on his own aircraft frequently or the manager of a restaurant to eat his own food.

How can we talk to our customers? It's easy. By walking around for a few minutes every day and making a point of stopping in a few patient rooms. By asking them about their care and the attitude of the staff. Ask them how long it takes to have a pain medication delivered and how hot the food is when it reaches their bedside. By spending a few minutes in the emergency room waiting room and asking whether or not the nursing staff is keeping them informed. By talking to the mother of a pediatric patient and asking about the quality of attention her child is receiving.

One CEO even goes so far as to copy his counterparts in fine hotels by putting a copy of a welcome greeting in each new patient's room and a special phone number for that patient to use to access the hospital CEO directly should there be a problem or a desire to single out a staff member for special praise. This hospital CEO has learned that the special phone line provides many opportunities to turn problems into positive stories about his hospital.

He tells the story of receiving a phone call from a patient one morning who was "bored." She requested some crochet needles and some yarn to keep her occupied while she waited nervously for surgery later in the day. She had no friends or relatives nearby. The CEO dispatched his secretary to a nearby K-Mart to purchase some needles and yarn. He then personally delivered them to the patient. Within hours, the story of the crochet needle delivery had reached the entire patient population and staff of the hospital. In all, the CEO invested $2.79 and several minutes of his personal time. The positive "advertising" created from that minute time investment is more powerful than thousands of dollars of media advertising. Why? Because it's personal.

On communicating with physicians

Communicating with physicians is an art form that some claim is beyond the abilities of hospital leaders, mortals that they are. I strongly disagree and believe it is quite possible to communicate effectively with 90 percent of physicians. The other ten percent are inhabitants of the "paranoid fringe" and no amount of communication, listening, or exhortation is going to reach them. Ignoring the paranoid fringe is the first lesson to learn in communicating with physicians.

One very effective way to communicate with physicians is to treat them like board members. Have enough courage to take them into your confidence and share information with them that they are not normally used to hearing. Hospital leaders willing to take some chances in communicating may be rewarded with new found respect among their physicians. The hospital CEO who shares the same operating information, including financial reports, with his medical staff that he shares with his board is a courageous communicator indeed.

One hospital CEO, facing a major employee layoff, announced the details of the impending layoff to physicians before telling the employees. For the first time, that group of physicians felt taken into management's confidence. Believe it or not, not one word about the impending layoff leaked to employees even though physicians had intimate knowledge of the details two weeks in advance. What is the moral here? It is trust, pure and simple. If hospital leaders have the courage to trust their physicians with confidential information they may be rewarded with a level of cooperation never before achieved.

Another way to communicate with physicians is the use of ad hoc groups. Some social scientists call this concensus building. John Kennedy was frequently accused by detractors of selecting a small group of supporters whenever he had a new program that he wanted to sell. Once the support group was convinced, he would widen the group of participants and let the original group sell the expanded group on the concept. The same concept works quite well with physicians.

Most hospital leaders have experienced extreme frustration in gaining acceptance for new ideas and concepts from their physicians. However, regardless of the idea or concept, hospital leaders can almost always find a small group of supporters with something to gain from the new idea. Using that group then to develop the concept and "sell" the idea to a wider group of physicians can work quite nicely. Of course, they might be accused of being a concensus builder just like John Kennedy, but what self respecting hospital leaders would mind that analogy?

One extremely effective model of physician communication was demonstrated by an inner city Chicago teaching hospital in the midst of its recent struggle for survival. The hospital's CEO and his four senior vice presidents each assigned themselves to the hospital's highest admitting physicians. They met frequently with the physicians, in the physicians' offices, and learned intimately the frustrations and the satisfactions which confronted their key physicians. In effect, this hospital's leadership group created a mentor relationship for key physicians. They were able to take constructive action on the physician concerns and strengthen the areas already satisfying their physicians and thereby opened a new and constructive form of communication. By the way, the CEO went one step further to insure that the improved communication level was sustained by making the satisfaction of the ten physicians part of the evaluation criteria for his senior vice presidents.

Another secret in communicating with physicians is to treat them like peers. Many "old style" hospital leaders have been intimidated in the past by physicians. Of course, there is good reason for this. Many physicians felt that the best way to get at a hospital CEO or his senior management was through "cocktail party" criticism with board members. Support of the leadership by the board can go a long way in doing away with this malarkey. Hospital leaders should feel comfortable in confronting physicians directly when needed. This is a new concept for some leaders, but one long overdue. It is a fact of hospital life that sometimes physicians pursue their own interests to the detriment of their hospital's interest. When that happens, hospital leaders should confront them and do what's necessary to protect their hospital's best interests, even if this means major conflicts with their physicians. Though painful, some hospital leaders believe this type of relationship may even engender a new respect for hospital leaders in the future.

Finally, there are always social opportunities for communicating with physicians. Sometimes, weak hospital leaders take this concept too far. For example, they think that having coffee and donuts with physicians in the lounge a couple of times a week is a great way of communicating. It can also be incredibly naive. Although there is nothing inherently wrong with the coffee and donut routine, it is not likely to sustain the hospital leader in the event of a major confrontation.

In summary, hospital leaders can communicate with their physicians in many ways. Treating them like trustees by sharing detailed information about the hospital is one way. Visiting them in their own office settings on occasion to solicit ideas about hospital services is another very fruitful way.

Communicating with employees

I once knew a hospital leader who was so incensed that a new nurse did not know his name that he completely lost his temper, grabbed her name tag, and proceeded to rip it off in the style of a general stripping a subordinate of his medals. Unforunately, the front of her new nurse's uniform was also ripped off, exposing her well-endowed bosom to several nearby staff members and patients. A pretty extreme example, but a true one nevertheless. The best way for hospital leaders to initiate communication and set the standards with employees is to participate in the orientation of new employees.

Hospital leaders, particularly the CEO, should let their employees know from the very beginning who they are and what they stand for. The simplest way to do this is for the CEO to participate by making the opening remarks in new employee orientation. This may only require half an hour or so every month, but is a reflection of the hospital leader's interest in new employees. The CEO should also use the new employee orientation as an opportunity to formally introduce his senior management. Some hospital leaders have long ago delegated orientating employees to education departments and personnel directors. This does not make the new employee orientation experience as productive as it could be. Those hospital leaders who have delegated this assignment away should reconsider.

Walking around is another way to communicate with employees. However, recognize the different qualities to walking around. Some hospital leaders make it a point to spend 5 or 10 minutes on a nursing unit or department several times a week talking with individual employees about their work experiences. This type of communicating time is quality time. Other hospital leaders approach walking around by speeding through the corridors smiling and waving but never stopping for even thirty seconds to actually talk with an employee. While this may contribute to keeping the hospital leader's weight under control, it does little to enhance communication. Management by walking around should not be considered a muscle building exercise. It should be considered a listening exercise. The more frequently it is done, the better hospital leaders understand the day to day joys and frustrations of their employees and managers.

"State of the Union" meetings are another good way to communicate with employees. Many hospital CEOs shun this approach as too much effort, but it is one of the best ways to keep employees informed about the present and future of their organization. Not only can the hospital CEO review the ups and downs of the past and present, but he can use "State of the Union" meetings to reinforce his vision of the hospital's future and to reinforce the corporate values which he and his senior executives espouse.

How often? Well, once a month is probably too much and once a year is probably not enough. Finding a happy medium of several meetings a year seems to be an excellent choice. By the way, the effectiveness of these meetings can be tremendously enhanced if the hospital CEO is willing to take questions from the employee audience following the formal presentation. This, of course, requires a certain commitment by the CEO to answer any and all questions as best he can. However, as many hospital leaders can attest, some of the most productive comments come as a result of dealing with rumors and questions from the audience rather than from the prepared presentation.

More employee contact

Sometimes, an employee ombudsman can be a useful vehicle if that position reports directly to the hospital CEO. Regardless of organization charts and chains of command, some employees cannot or will not express concerns to their supervisors. Indeed, sometimes their concerns deal directly with how they are treated by their supervisors. An employee ombudsman can give employees a direct channel to the hospital CEO, sometimes necessary to resolve issues. Members of middle management may be threatened by this position. What is important is not who and why middle management gets threatened, but that the effectiveness of communication between employees and hospital leader is accomplished. Correctly structured, the employee ombudsman position can successfully achieve this goal.

Another successful approach used by several hospitals is the monthly briefing with "selected" employees. This technique goes under different descriptions from informally selected employees for "coffee hours" with the hospital CEO to other more formally defined small group meetings with hospital leaders. The essential concept here is to select employees from various work units to get a more detailed briefing on the activities of the hospital and upcoming activities.

Some hospital leaders will argue that this represents a company union. Nonsense. If the employees are picked on a voluntary basis and hospital leaders avoid discussing wages and working conditions, this forum can be used as an extremely effective technique for communicating with employees. It provides an opportunity to bring to the surface issues which have not received adequate attention through the formal management ranks. It requires the commitment of several hours a month from hospital leaders for direct employee conversation and a commitment to resolve surfaced issues. It is a commitment worth every minute of the time invested.

How about communicating pay raises and bonuses? The way in which the hospital announces pay raises is a good indicator of the value its leaders place on personal communication. Is there a general verbal announcement made by the CEO to the management staff, who then communicate it verbally to employees? Or does the CEO take the time and effort to communicate directly with each employee with a personal letter to his home? There is no substitute for a direct communication from the hospital CEO to every employee, thanking them for their efforts which made the pay raise possible.

Personal letters should be hand signed or the value of the personal communication is greatly diminished. Even a hospital leader with 1,500 employees can sign personal letters of this nature in a few hours. And how about bonuses? Some hospitals are fortunate enough to be able to grant an employee bonus, but fail to gain maximum impact by communicating it poorly. Is the bonus merely added onto the last paycheck of the year? Or, is it sent with a personalized Christmas card, signed by the hospital CEO? Even more impressive is giving a cash bonus, like a $100 bill, rather than a cold and impersonal check. It is a shame to have hospitals lose the impact of giving a bonus merely because of poor communication.

Communicating with the community

How do hospital leaders get the most out of communicating with their community? Should they constantly be on the speaking circuit of Rotary and Kiwanis? Should they be members of those groups to informally rub elbows with other community leaders? There is no one answer to this question. Communities and hospitals vary greatly. Hospital leaders vary greatly in their communication skills in front of groups and media. Here are a few suggestions.

Dealing with the media is always a challenge. Newspaper editors and television newscasters employ different techniques for expressing their differing points of view. Cultivating the local newspaper is an extremely important task of the hospital CEO. Whether small town or large, the newspaper has much to say about the content and slant of coverage for the leader's hospital. A good relationship with the local paper can result in better coverage of hospital events and fairer coverage in times of conflict with unions, lawsuits, and other difficult situations. Hospital leaders should take the time to cultivate the best possible relationship with local newspapers.

Television is another matter. Television tells stories in a few seconds. There is no time for elaboration or explanation. There is also no guarantee about what gets edited before air time. Use television for noteworthy news events, but pull back in the event of controversy. Union organizing and lawsuits become sensationalized stories by television. Although the hospital leader may make an elegant case for his hospital's point of view, it may very well end up on the editor's chopping block. Therefore, it is better to stay away from television with controversial events while reporting the story to the newspaper in a positive way.

Community leaders are a largely untapped resource for hospital leaders. Several midwest CEOs make a point of inviting community leaders to the hospital once a year for a tour with the senior management and a "State of the Union" address. This gives community leaders an opportunity to ask questions about the hospital's progress and plans, and gives the hospital leaders a tremendous opportunity to "sell" their programs to people who matter. It is helpful to bring two types of leaders into these types of sessions. One type of community leader is self-evident. They are the individuals who run the major corporations and who head the major interest groups. The other group is more subtle. They are the opinion leaders, the folks who talk with large numbers of community residents. These types of individuals are the successful real estate salesmen, the car dealers, the beauty shop operators, and the retail store owners and managers. They are just as important, if not more important, in getting the message out to the community about what the hospital is doing and planning for the future.

Another excellent vehicle of communication with the community is to give hospital related speeches to community groups. Service clubs, church groups, and civic groups are always looking for good speakers. A well executed presentation can work wonders to inform the community about the hospital's present and future outlook. It also gives large numbers of individuals an opportunity to ask questions and identify areas of dissatisfaction. Beware, however; hospital leaders can go overboard on the speaking circuit. The CEO has to be the judge of how much and what format is appropriate for his community. Members of the senior management and members of the medical staff can be very effective presenters. Direct communication with civic groups and community leaders is a very effective tool in telling the hospital story to the community.

To be most effective, leaders must do it personally. There is no substitute for the hospital's CEO and senior management talking to patients. There is no substitute for the leaders talking with employees, physicians, and the community. Personal contact with the leaders sets the tone for everyone else. If they can take the time, so can their middle managers, and their staff. Resist delegating communication. Do it yourself and make it personal.

CHAPTER FOUR

Details, Details, Details

MUCH HAS BEEN WRITTEN lately in popular management books about the value of paying attention to details. Remember the references in *A Passion For Excellence* about chicken wing hairs? Frank Purdue, the east coast chicken king, is a notable example of an organization leader paying attention to detail. Mr. Purdue recognized that consumers do not appreciate the presence of "feather hair" on fresh chicken wings. He even went to the trouble of building a gigantic machine, powered by a 727 jet engine, to remove chicken wing hairs so that his customers would not begin to question the quality of his chicken due to a few hairy wings.

In a hospital setting, details are everything. A lack of attention to detail by hospital staff can lead patients to conclude that they are getting poor quality patient care. Hospital leaders, both CEOs and senior managers, need to pay much closer attention to details. They need to pay attention personally, while instilling a passion for attention to detail in their supervisory staff and employees. Some hospital leaders get defensive when you talk about the importance of attention to detail. They self-righteously point out that attention to detail is for employees. Perhaps that is because they do not talk much about details in business or hospital administration schools.

Hospitals need a lot of work in the area of attention to detail. The same hospital leaders who get defensive about whose job attention to detail is, are probably the same executives whose patients and visitors are greeted by a "Gravel Gertie" receptionist as their first impression, and a "Bank Teller" cashier's window in the hospital lobby as their last impression. First and last impressions are the end points. The thousands of details in between are what hospital leaders need to focus their energies on. Jan Carlson, President of SAS Airlines, described details as "moments of truth." He once observed, "We have 50,000 moments of truth out there every day." A moment of truth by Carlson's definition is an episode in which a customer comes in contact with any aspect of the company, however remote, and thereby has an opportunity to form an impression.[8] It would be impossible to cover good and bad examples of the thousands of details experienced in our hospitals today. What follows are a few examples of the best and worst hospital "moments of truth."

Down with plastic dinnerware

The admitting process is a good place to start when observing attention to detail. In some hospitals, it is a gauntlet designed for the convenience of insurance companies and hospital computer operators, rather than an experience intended to create a good first impression on our customers. There are exceptions, however. An impressive Memphis hospital has created a system whereby patients are greeted at the lobby entrance by a doorman and taken directly to their room. They are introduced to the room amenities and systems such as the nurse call lights, television controls, showers.[9] Then, a representative of the admitting department comes to the room to take care of the "paper work" associated with admission. This hospital truly understands the importance of creating a positive first impression for its customers. It's a program worth emulating.

Hospitals have much to learn from hotels when it comes to paying attention to amenity details. It never ceases to amaze some of our customers that, in spite of paying extremely high daily room rates, they still get a measly one ounce bar of soap and a towel capable only of drying a small portion of one's body. A few, very few indeed, hospitals are beginning to understand the importance of creating an "amenities kit" worthy of the price our customers pay for their hospital rooms. They are throwing out the cheap plastic cups, the flimsy combs, and the tiny kleenex boxes suitable only for newborn infants.

It's impossible to leave a discussion of patient details without touching on the use of disposables in hospitals. Although I certainly would not advocate returning to the reusing and sharping of syringe needles, it is safe to say hospitals have gotten carried away with the use of cheap plastic disposable items in non-clinical areas. A case in point is water pitchers. In many hospitals, patients are expected to make due with a cheap plastic disposable water pitcher. The two main features of these water pitchers are that they keep ice water cold only for an hour or two and that they then sweat all over the bedside stand creating a puddle of water to slip on when a patient needs to get out of bed. Hospitals should invest in high quality thermal water pitchers that work well for years and actually keep ice cold for six to eight hours. They also cost less in the long run than the disposable ones in use in many hospitals.

We also must touch on the rising use of disposables by food service departments in hospitals. This is a disgrace. Having patients eat off styrofoam plates, drink their beverages from plastic cups, and try to cut their food with plastic knifes and forks say how little attention those hospitals pay to practical patient details. Not only does the use of cheap disposables give a poor quality impression, they cost more than the use of reusable stainless steel dinnerware and "real" plates, glasses, and cups.

Not only is it important what the patients eat off of, the quality and type of the food they eat is equally important. When food is served, it should be hot, be tasteful, and be what the patient ordered. But paying attention to details goes far beyond the quality and presentation of the food. The design of menus should be kept in mind as well. Patients' circumstances are especially important. An excellent example of circumstance inattention is serving peas to post surgery patients. Everyone knows that peas cause gas, and gas is painful for post surgery patients. An examination of the menus provided to post surgery patients in many hospitals will likely discover gas-causing foods on the menu. Before laughing, check out your own menu!

How about mattresses and pillows? Pillows and mattresses would be a lot more comfortable if hospital CEOs and their senior management had to spend six or seven days in bed once in a while in their own hospitals. One progressive Massachusetts hospital makes it part of the housekeeper's room changing routine to check comfort by getting into bed and testing all mattresses and pillows before the room is placed back in service after a patient's discharge.

Mattresses and pillows that fail the "comfort test" are immediately taken out of service and replaced.

An interesting hotel concept implemented by a Wisconsin hospital is a free patient and family pick-up and delivery service. It's called "Patient Express" and is modeled after hotel transport vans which are used in major cities and airports throughout the country. The Patient Express service is available free of charge to patients needing to get to and from the hospital. It is occasionally used for bringing visitors to the hospital who are unable to get there through any other public transportation systems. Not only does this service project an aura of caring to the community—it actually increased the outpatient business in several hospital departments like physical therapy.

Physicians can also be extremely helpful in paying attention to patient details if appropriately motivated. For example, a progressive group of anesthesiologists in Minnesota hand out Sony Walkman cassette players to all of their patients awaiting surgery. The music eases the anxiety of waiting, and lets the patient know that physicians really care about their comfort.

Just about every department in hospitals could pay more attention to patient details, even the business office. Business offices could begin by looking at two details of tremendous importance to patients. The first is the language used on hospital bills. They must ask themselves whether the language used to describe the various charge items are written in "computerese" and medical terminology only a physician could understand. If so, they would do their customers a great favor by changing the terminology and making it simple enough so that their customers could understand it. They might find they get fewer questions on their bills if they did so.

Another detail which many business offices do not pay attention to is sending bills to deceased patients. Imagine this scenario. You are a 69-year-old wife who has just lost your husband of 43 years. Prior to his death, he spent three weeks in a hospital and finally succumbed to a terminal illness. Somehow, with the help of your family you were able to get through the funeral arrangements for your beloved husband. Then, a week later, you receive a bill from your husband's hospital, addressed to him, for $20,000. The first thought that crosses your mind is how cold and heartless that hospital must be to send a bill to a deceased person, particularly since that person died in their facility. Sound like a "horror story"? Better check your own business office to see how they send bills to deceased patients.

Even hospitals that sucessfully pay attention to detail are not perfect. The use of a patient ombudsman system can help address the inevitable problems that arise, even in a well-led hospital.

A patient ombudsmen can resolve problems and identify areas where the hospital could perform better for its customers. The position is similar to a concierge's position used by fine hotels. One Wisconsin hospital has carried the patient ombudsmen concept one giant step further than most hospitals. They have recognized that part of the value in having a patient ombudsmen is being able to give immediate relief to patient problems. Therefore, instead of having the patient ombudsmen fill out five forms and obtain permission from the head nurse, department director and two vice presidents before resolving a minor problem, she carries a checkbook and the authority to use it.

For example, when patients lose a contact lens, their dentures are damaged, or an item of clothing is lost the patient ombudsmen immediately writes out a check at the bedside to compensate the patients for the loss. No arguments, no forms in triplicate, just immediate action. This hospital found that in the course of a year very little money was expended by utilizing this approach. However, the fact that the ombudsmen could issue a check immediately enhanced the credibility and the effectiveness of the position.

Squeaky wheels and coffee stains

The design, maintenance, and appearance of our hospitals can either promote or detract from a hospital's ability to project a caring and competent image to their customers. The first set of opportunities are on the access roads and parking lots of hospitals. Are the signs large enough to be read and easily understood by people trying to find the hospital? Many times architects and sign designers care more about the elegance of the design on paper than the practical value of their signs when they are in place. Attention should also be paid to the grooming of the sidewalks and the grounds. This is a safety as well as aesthetic issue. Well-kept grounds, sidewalks, and access roads look better and cause fewer falls on the hospital property. This is particularly important during the winter months when hospitals should be watchful that there is no ice or snow on roadways or sidewalks.

Once inside the building, patients and visitors have hundreds of cues about the hospital's attention to detail. One is the cleanliness of facilities, particularly high traffic areas like lobbies, elevators, and waiting rooms. Also, clinical areas are of much importance to patients and visitors. For example, when patients go into a floroscope room in x-ray they may become concerned if they see heavy electrical cables lying about the floor or in a disorderly mess on the walls or ceiling. Even worse, they may become dismayed if ceiling tiles are missing while they are laying flat on their back with nothing else to look at but the empty space where the ceiling tiles should have been replaced after a maintenance engineer adjusted the plumbing.

Another good place to look at ceilings is in the operating rooms. With the emphasis on spinal anesthesia and local anesthesia, many patients are "awake" during surgery. What do they see? In some hospitals they see an eclectic combination of high tech anesthesia machines and twenty-year-old instrument stands. They might also see crude handwritten signs done in magic marker and covered with blue x-ray film taped to the wall with yellowed surgery tape. I do not know what it is about blue x-ray film, but hospital employees seem to love using it as a cover for paper signs. That is not the kind of symbol which stimulates confidence in our customers.

In the patient rooms, facility details are also important. Shower pressure and how long it takes to get hot water are very important to our patients. If the chief engineer had to take a shower under a "dribbling" shower head, he might get more passionate about checking them more frequently for mineral deposits which obstruct the spray jets. If he had to wait ten minutes for hot water in the shower after being bedridden for a week he might get a lot more interested in checking hot water delivery to the customers' rooms.

Hospitals, even small ones, have millions of dollars invested in their buildings and equipment. For the most part, they take good care of the sophisticated equipment and building systems, but do not do as good a job when it comes to small equipment items related to patients. I know of one hospital that thought it was doing a big favor for its ICU patients by purchasing bedside radios. They purchased the cheapest portables they could find. After several months, those radios were being held together by rubber bands and surgical tape because they had been frequently knocked off the bedside stands. They finally got better radios when a patient requested to be transferred to another hospital because he was afraid that his heart monitor was as cheap as the bedside radio.

Noise is also an important detail consideration. Have you ever thought about how distracting it is for patients to listen to the squeaky wheels of the countless carts used in hospitals? How about ice machine compressors that are not properly adjusted and keep patients up all night? Or the PA system that startles patients and staff alike because its volume control is out of adjustment? Noise may not be a "big executive" concern, but it should be because patients' rest and recovery problems are compounded when it is neglected.

Patients cannot evaluate the efficiency of a CT scanner. But they can and do get worried if equipment they use does not work. Think how frustrated a patient gets when the TV controls do not work right. Besides getting frustrated, he might begin drawing conclusions about the quality of care being poor if the hospital cannot even make a simple TV control work properly.

A successful airline executive once observed that airline customers formed negative impressions about aircraft maintenance if they found coffee stains on their seat back tray. Hospitals that do not pay enough attention to detail create the same set of worries in their customers if their facilities and equipment are not maintained superbly.

Baseball caps belong on TV nurses only

It is fascinating to see the range of staff attire in hospitals. On one extreme, you can observe an expensively tailored suit on an executive or physician, and on the other extreme observe a housekeeper or food service worker in tattered blue jeans. Like coffee stains on airline seat trays, our customers draw conclusions about the quality of our hospitals from attire and physical appearance of hospital staffs. In the rush to be considered flexible employers, some hospitals have gone too far and lowered appearance standards too much. It is a shame to see blue jeans in a professional setting. Track shoes and clogs are equally unimpressive. Who wants to see a nurse in a baseball cap or an emergency room physician in sandals and a Hawaiian shirt? It may be good enough for "St. Elsewhere," but not in a well-led hospital.

Uniforms should always be cleaned and pressed. Shoes should be polished. Hair and nails should be well cared for. It is a poor reflection of the hospital's leadership if their staff looks sloppy and unprofessional. You do not see any slobs working in McDonald's, Sears, or Delta Airlines. You should not see them in hospitals either, but you do. They do not teach you to look for dirty fingernails in MHA programs. However, good leaders should have enough common sense and high enough personal standards that they learn to do that all by themselves.

It is also important for hospital leaders to give high priority to details which are important to their employees. For example, employee lounges express the hospital leaders' commitment to their staff. Are they as beautifully furnished as the hospital lobby and spotlessly clean as the operating rooms? If they are not, it means that hospital leaders are not paying as much attention to their staff as they are to the public. That level of indifference indicates poor leadership.

Two other details employees take seriously are food and parking lots. Hospitals should provide excellent quality and variety of food to all three shifts. Special attention needs to be paid to the night shift. One midwest hospital's senior management goes to the time and trouble to come in several times a year and on holidays to serve a special gourmet meal to night shift employees. A small detail perhaps, but one much appreciated by the "forgotten" shift. With reference to parking lots, be sure that there are enough spaces and that they are shoveled properly when it snows. For hospitals in cold climates, a nice touch is to make available jump-starts on those cold winter nights when the 3-11 and 11-7 shifts can't get their frozen cars going.

If hospital leaders want their employees to pay attention to detail, then those same leaders should pay attention to the details which matter most to employees. Anything less is leadership hypocrisy.

Chicken wing lessons

Perceptions about a hospital and its leaders are the cumulation of our customers interpreting hundreds and perhaps thousands of details. Patients may not be able to evaluate the elegance of our financial control system; however, they are well prepared to judge the quality of the food and the appearance of our employees. It is the job of hospital leaders to establish the importance of paying attention to details in everyone's mind. That means physicians, managers, auxiliary members, and employees. Hospitals that pay attention to details can clearly differentiate themselves in the market place and can compete effectively even with institutions of much larger size.

If Frank Purdue can worry about the hair on chicken wings, hospital leaders too can put a great deal more energy in the details that matter to their customers.

CHAPTER FIVE

Organization: Keep It Simple

RAY KROC, founder of McDonald's, had a longstanding theory of organization design: "less is more." It is too bad Mr. Kroc did not spend some of his time consulting for the hospital industry. There are too many managers and too few leaders in hospitals. We have fooled ourselves into believing that more managers mean better outcomes. In fact, the opposite may be true. The old saying about too many chiefs and not enough Indians rings true for hospitals. We have over-invested in managerial layers and staff positions, and have lost touch with the outcomes our organization should produce. Peter Drucker is said to have remarked that "most of what we call management consists of making it difficult for people to get their work done." It follows that less management may mean more effectiveness.

With rare exceptions, America's best-run companies practice the "less is more" approach. Dana Corporation, Johnson and Johnson, and Wal-Mart have lean corporate organizations. Their leaders understand the value of listening to their customers without "middle management" interference. Automobile companies are also beginning to trim their numbers in middle management to become more competitive with the Japanese.

Perhaps one of the most fundamental questions facing a hospital CEO is how best to design his organization for effectiveness. A step in the right direction is to reduce the size of his management staff by one-third and cut the number of organization layers in half. As the dust settles, the work of the hospital organization—taking care of sick people—still gets done and probably more effectively.

Elimination of organization layers

The hospital CEO is responsible for ensuring that as many sick people as possible get better while under his or her institution's care. This means that hospital CEOs should be accountable for running their organization, rather than being the "outside person," which is currently in vogue. Many hospitals have gotten carried away with the pyramidal structure of organization, which essentially delegates the running of the hospital to subordinates so the CEO can concentrate on external affairs. It is not uncommon to find three to five managerial layers between the chief executive officer and the hourly hospital employees. Figure 2 is a typical hospital organization. In some larger hospitals, there are even more layers. Do we really need all of these middle managers?

A small to medium size hospital (300 beds or under) can utilize a two-layer organization very effectively. This means doing without a chief operating officer and several other middle managerial levels. If the hospital CEO sees his job as that of running the organization first, and interfacing with the external environment second, this type of organizational structure will work. It is only necessary to have

FIGURE 2

TYPICAL HOSPITAL TABLE OF ORGANIZATION

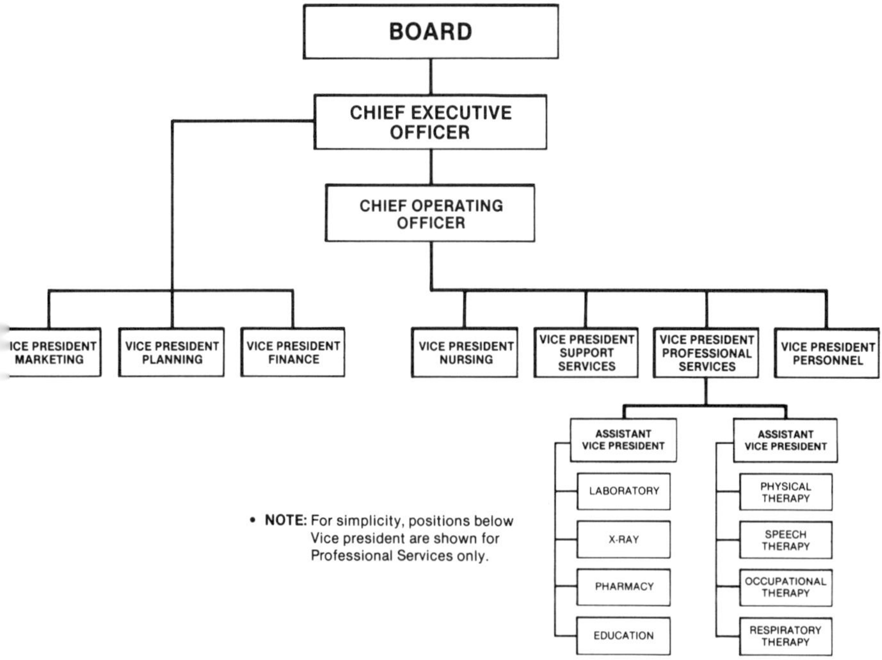

• **NOTE:** For simplicity, positions below Vice president are shown for Professional Services only.

department heads and vice presidents as the two layers that are absolutely essential in a small to medium-sized hospital.

More and more CEOs are getting away from knowing their hospital. They are spending more time on community boards, network committees, and hospital association committees. Many CEOs would have to admit that their "outside" activities do little, if anything, to contribute to their hospital's success. Why do they do it then? Because of the "herd" mentality of many hospital CEOs. They do it because other CEOs do it, not because of inherent value. Interesting to note is that some CEOs lose their jobs after taking leadership roles in state and national hospital organizations. Perhaps they simply lose touch with their organizations. Unfortunately, too many CEOs are losing touch because of the time they spend on "external affairs."

Let's stop overdoing staff positions

Hospitals have too many staff positions. The growth in vice presidential level positions like marketing and planning is a good example. Many hospital leaders think that hiring a vice president of marketing is the instant pathway to success. Many also believe that having a vice president of planning relieves them of the responsibility of planning. Some hospital leaders think that having a vice president of management information services will produce better outcomes. Nothing could be farther from the truth.

The hospital CEO and his senior management should be the marketers and the planners for their organization. Not all staff positions are bad. Even a conservative like myself would admit that financial and personnel executives are necessary staff positions. However, when it comes to planning and marketing, there is no substitute for having the CEO and senior management assume these responsibilities for their organization. Likewise, we are producing far too much data for most hospitals to use. Doing away with the information services position might enhance the organization's performance rather than inhibit it. All of the responsibilities currently being performed by "staffers" could be reassigned to the service line managers, with better accountability and better results.

Some thoughts about nursing organizations

Nursing organizations are fertile ground for organizational obesity. The typical hospital nursing organization has more layers than the rest of the organization put together. Not unknown is the pyramid that starts with charge or assistant head nurses, moves up to head nurse, then up again to assistant nursing director, then further still to associate director, and finally to director of nursing. Sometimes, there are even assistant administrators (or vice presidents) above the director of nursing. That adds up to six layers of bureaucracy in nursing. Figure 3 represents a typical nursing organization in a medium-sized hospital.

This type of bureaucracy stems from a lack of insight by many hospital CEOs about the job of head nurse. Head nurse positions should be equivalent in status and responsibility to other department heads. Treating head nurses as second class managers is hypocritical. In most hospitals, head nurses have the direct responsibility of taking care of our patients, our customers, but are not given the equivalent status of a department head. It is ridiculous to relegate head nurses to a status lower than the head of the physical therapy or engineering department.

FIGURE 3

TYPICAL NURSING DEPARTMENT TABLE OF ORGANIZATION

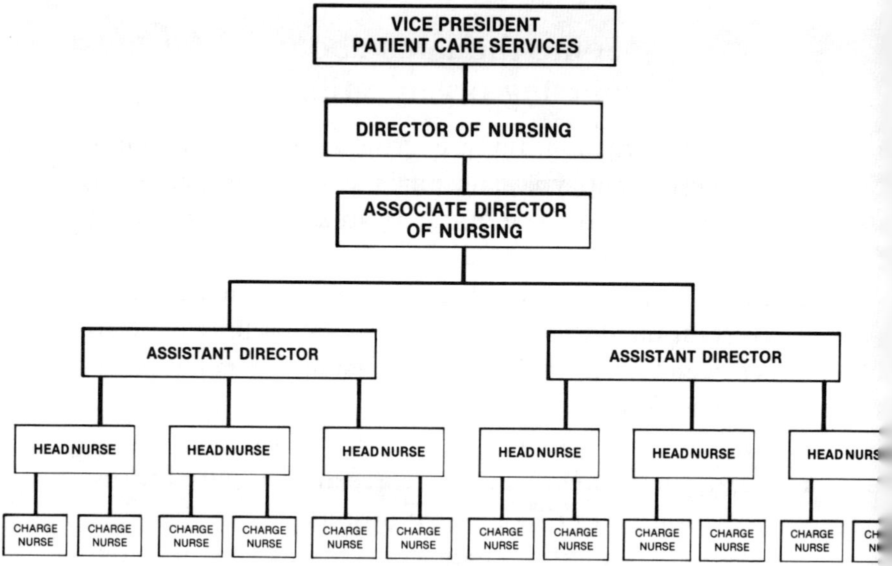

Head nurses should be considered department heads. One administrative person above them is all that is necessary, even in a large hospital. For this type of leaned-out nursing organization to take place, the hospital CEO must embrace the concept of having head nurses as department heads. Why are only a few hospitals embracing this concept? Maybe they are paying too much attention to their vice presidents of nursing and not enough attention to common sense.

Administrative staff assignments

There is great variation in departmental assignments among hospital administrative staffs. Often, a vice president is in charge of a mixture of unrelated departments. Sometimes this is done to accommodate the strengths, or weaknesses, of individual executives. Sometimes this is done for reasons of organization inertia. "That's the way we have always done it" is the key phrase for organization design in some hospitals.

Four or fewer vice presidents are an optimal size staff for hospitals of 100 to 300 beds, the majority of hospitals in the United States. The four are: professional services, support services, finance, and nursing. Support services and finance, and nursing and professional services can sometimes be combined, depending on the strengths of the individuals in those positions. It makes sense to organize hospital administrative staffs along these functional lines. Some leaders say that this approach is somewhat old-fashioned. But it works very well in most hospitals and it provides for internal growth. The support services position provides excellent training for the professional services position, while the nursing, finance, and professional services positions provide excellent training for the CEO position, depending on the individuals and organization's needs.

A two-layer lean organization

A two-layer organization, illustrated in Figure 4, would easily serve a hospital of up to 300 beds. Note the absence of staff positions like planning and marketing. These duties are part of the CEO and vice president positions. Note also that several department head positions report directly to the CEO, like personnel and community relations. This is a simple, lean organization that works.

A word about senior management

To make a simple and lean hospital organization work requires the recruitment or development of assistant administrators or vice presidents who have capabilities above what is normally found in hospitals. It requires senior managers who are comfortable with and capable of handling staff work like planning and marketing. It also requires a CEO who is comfortable and capable in these areas.

These people are not that common in the hospital industry, but they do exist. Most hospitals have come to depend so much on staffers that the vice president and CEOs cannot begin to write a long-range plan or develop and execute a marketing strategy. Observers of management are beginning to describe the dismantling of planning departments in large business firms. We are going to see the same thing happen in hospitals.

The success of implementing a simpler and leaner hospital organization depends on recruiting, training and retaining senior managers who are capable of handling staff functions for their own areas of responsibility.

FIGURE 4

SIMPLIFIED HOSPITAL TABLE OF ORGANIZATION

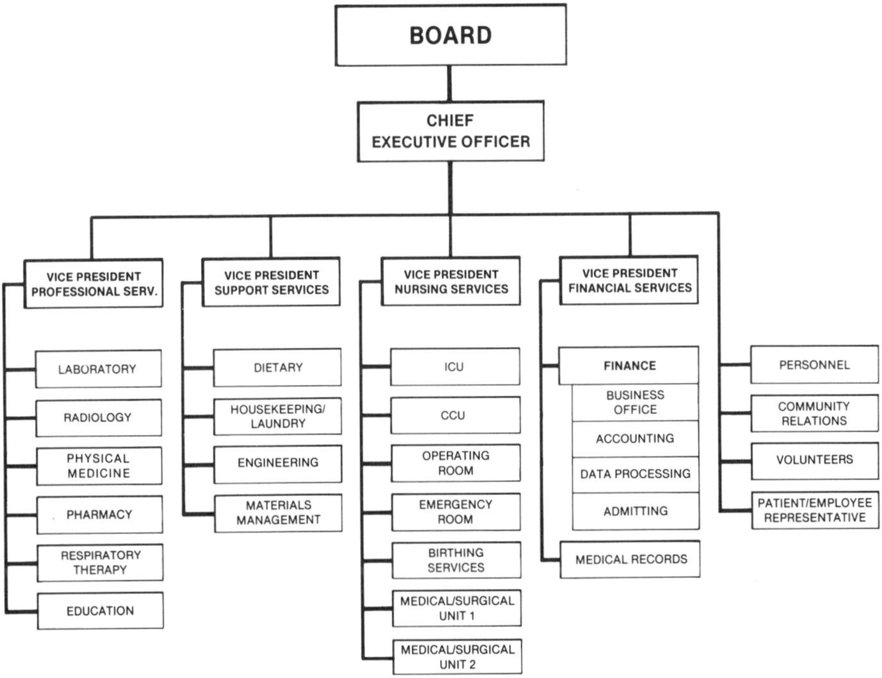

Some concluding thoughts

One of the best ways a CEO can improve the effectiveness of his hospital is to reduce the ranks of middle management. Assuming that the hospital is under 300 beds–80 percent of hospitals in this country are–it is possible to reduce the number of organization layers to two without sacrificing the quality of management. It requires a commitment on the part of the CEO to really know his or her hospital better than most leaders do. Communication will be easier, management will require less financial resources, and ultimately the patients will be better served because the leaders will be more in touch with their organizations. It is tough to do, but once accomplished, leaders will never return to the old five-layer pyramids.

PART TWO

LEADING THE HOSPITAL

CHAPTER SIX

Know Your Hospital

PETER DRUCKER once remarked that one of the most important things an organization can do is to determine what business it is in. To carry his thought one step further, hospital leaders should remember they are in the patient care business, not the holding company business nor the hospital association committee business nor the vertical integration business.

One of the biggest problems in hospitals is that leaders do not know enough about what is going on in their own organizations. To be effective, hospital leaders must pay more attention to the outcomes produced in their organization. This may come at the expense of a few Rotary meetings and committee memberships with state hospital associations. Hospital leaders are responsible for overseeing the operation of the entire hospital. The CEO is ultimately responsible for everything, and his senior managers are responsible for the outcomes produced in their areas of responsibility.

Knowing what is going on is essential to provide good leadership in hospital operations. A working definition of operations in a hospital is a department's product or service. In physical therapy, it is whether a stroke patient can satisfactorily return to activities of daily living after treatments. In housekeeping, it is whether the environment is sparkling clean. Each and every department in a hospital produces a product or service that has a definitive outcome. There are qualitative and quantitative outcomes that, taken in their entirety, can be described as the operation of a hospital.

Hospital leaders are responsible for instilling in their department heads and ultimately their employees the importance of effective operations. The hospital leaders' job is also to establish the overall operating standards for their institution, both quantitative and qualitative. Each department has an outcome and the hospital leaders responsible for those departments should see to it that definitive performance standards are established. This is the real nitty-gritty aspect of hospital leadership. It means rolling up sleeves to determine whether or not the laboratory is producing fast and accurate lab results, whether the operating room infection rate is within acceptable limits, and whether pulmonary care treatments are enhancing the recovery of critically ill patients.

The standards that hospital leaders set for their various departments are a reflection of themselves. When standards are set too high they will never be achieved, and poor morale and employee discouragement are sure to follow. When they are set too low, quality of care is not optimized. When there are no standards set, as is the case in some hospitals, the operations of the facility will drop to the lowest level allowing it to merely get by. In these days of increasing competition, hospitals that practice that sort of laissez faire standard setting will undoubtedly perish.

Knowing what to monitor

The second job of leadership in operations is knowing what to monitor and how frequently to monitor it. A CEO in a Chicago area hospital has created a superb monitoring system to track the operations from various departments within his hospital. His vice presidents must review the identified operating indicators on a monthly basis and explain any departures from the norm. It is a system that works somewhat like monitoring the financial operations; however, the indicators are operational in nature rather than financial. This well-defined accountability system for operations keeps managers focused on what is important to produce positive outcomes for patients.

Identifying what to monitor can be divided into two categories. Quantitative outcomes are quite easy to identify for well-informed hospital leaders. Each department has several quantitative outcomes that should be observed closely to monitor the department's effectiveness. Examples of quantitative standards: turnaround time for laboratory STAT requests, repeat rate for x-ray exams, medication error rates, time delays for answering patient call lights. The hospital leaders' job is to identify what is important for the patients in each hospital department. Once identified, standards must be set and department heads held accountable for meeting those standards on a continuous basis. This requires the vice presidential level leaders to become intimately familiar with the departments within their responsibility. This has not been the trend in recent years in hospital administration.

Vice presidents and assistant administrators tend to think of themselves as "big executives" and many find it beneath themselves to spend time in the trenches learning the intimate details of the departments they supervise. Some are so anxious to become CEOs that they consider it a waste of time to learn how long it takes to run a blood gas exam or how difficult speech therapy work is with an acute stroke patient.

This elitist attitude must change if hospital leaders are going to be successful. Vice presidents and assistant administrators must get down to the basic level and learn in great detail the operations of the departments they supervise.

There are many qualitative outcomes to be monitored in hospitals as well. Though a little more difficult, qualitative outcomes can be measured almost as well as quantitative outcomes. Essentially, we are talking about attitudinal issues. Are we solicitous for patient comfort when we draw blood? Are we awakening patients at 5 a.m. to weigh them simply because of physician rounding habits? Are we taking good care of family members who are interested in condition reports on patients? These qualitative outcomes can be measured with a statistically significant questionnaire that's administered routinely.

Statistically significant does not mean handing out "comment cards" on discharge. I mean routinely surveying a statistically significant population and categorizing their responses to get a true picture of the adequacy of services delivered. Many good programs are on the market today to accomplish this objective and I would encourage any hospital leader who is still using the old "comment card" system to abandon it and initiate a system using a statistically significant sample.

Defining operational standards

As stated earlier, hospital leaders must set the standards in the departments for which they are responsible. The CEO is responsible for setting the standards for his senior managers. These standards may be set in terms of financial performance, operational performance and customer relations performance. The senior managers are subsequently responsible for setting the standards in their departments.

For service departments like dietary, the vice president or assistant administrator in charge of support services should make certain the hospital is serving hot, attractive bedside meals which are of high quality. They should notice such details as whether or not the food is served on disposable dinnerware versus china and how patients perceive the meals, rather than how good the meals look and taste within the walls of the dietary department.

For clinical departments, the vice president or assistant administrator in charge of professional services should observe and set standards for things like infection rates in the operating room and turnaround time standards for laboratory exams. Familiarity with the operation of each department is important so operating standards can be comfortably set. Operating standards need to be articulated to the department managers and a monitoring system needs to be established so that feedback is provided on a regular basis.

Further, hospital leaders are responsible for establishing appropriate policies, procedures and training programs to ensure that all employees fully understand the standards and are able to accomplish them. Again, it is the job of hospital leaders to judge whether the policies are adequate, the equipment used to produce outcomes is satisfactory, and that training programs actually accomplish the intended results. Also, hospital leaders must be aware that standards need to be thoroughly evaluated on a timely basis. Several years ago, the standard for producing a blood gas measurement was approximately 30 minutes. The technology has changed significantly in the past several years, and an acceptable time for producing a blood gas currently would be no more than 5 minutes. It is the hospital leader's job to be familiar with changes in technology and update the standards.

Where are the senior managers going to get all the time to become familiar enough with their departments to set standards and then to monitor them? One way they can find the time is to attend fewer outside meetings. They can probably go to fewer meetings within the hospital as well. Next, they might want to take a look at their own work ethic. Vice president level executives in industry often work 10 to 16 hours a day. We need more of that kind of work ethic among hospital senior managers. Higher levels of energy and passion will go a long way in accomplishing better results for operating departments within hospitals.

Monitoring techniques

Hundreds of books have been written on techniques for monitoring operations. I would suggest a few simple techniques rooted more in common sense than esoteric management methods. First, hospital leaders should use their eyes and ears daily. Daily observations and questions asked of physicians, staff members, and most importantly patients are the strongest possible monitoring technique. Questions should stimulate probes on a positive and negative basis. The major assumption in utilizing this technique is that hospital leaders get around sufficiently in their own areas of responsibility to make daily observations and that they take the time to follow up on them. This requires a commitment to be present in hospital departments more often than is sometimes practiced by hospital leaders.

Another technique is "the random audit technique." This means that hospital leaders should show up on off shifts occasionally and make firsthand observations about the quality of food, the attentiveness of nursing staff, and the efficiency of the engineering department. Another aspect of random auditing: select a report, perhaps an incident report, and trace it back to its source by questioning each and every staff member and physician involved in the incident. Subordinates may sometimes confuse this approach with a lack of trust. However, an enlightened leader sees this technique as a way to ensure credibility up and down the organization.

A hospital leader can also thoroughly review monthly reports generated by the leader's department heads. These can be a combination of financial and operating reports structured to focus on the key operating and financial standards for the departments.

Follow-up

One of the most important aspects of monitoring operations is the follow-up. The effective monitoring of operations must always include follow-up when operations problems are discovered. Those problems that recur, such as difficulties with housekeeping during the winter months and increased medication error rates with the introduction of new nurses, can be anticipated and prevented by a leader who is well organized.

When operating problems of a non-recurring nature are discovered, effective leaders deal with them quickly and completely. One of the most important characteristics of an effective leader is persistence. Persistent leaders keep the number of operating problems in their areas of responsibility to a minimum, instilling in their line managers the notion that operations in their departments are their own responsibility.

Persistence among hospital leaders cannot be overemphasized. Sometimes problems cannot be resolved, regardless of the amount of time, energy, and money expended. For example, it is impossible to totally eliminate the possibility of medication errors in a hospital environment. However, with persistence it is possible to reduce the possibility of these errors to a minimum. It requires the commitment of pharmacists and nursing staff to develop the necessary in-service programs and systems to ensure accurate delivery of medication to the patients.

Planning ahead

The final responsibility in monitoring operations by hospital leaders is to plan ahead. Feedback mechanisms should identify patterns and trends. Incident reports can be used to identify trends in medication errors that generate a series of in-service programs or system changes to reduce possible errors. Monitoring operations requires constant vigilance and analysis on the part of hospital leaders. A passion for fine tuning operations and making incremental improvements in a thousand different areas is also needed.

A new concept of leadership

Who would have thought that being a CEO or a vice president in a hospital meant checking on the temperature of the coffee when it is delivered to the patient's bedside? Who would have thought that being a "big executive" meant finding out whether or not the receptionist is well-informed and friendly as she greets visitors and family members? These "leadership" skills are not taught in business or hospital administration school. But they are important.

Leaders in hospitals should certainly worry about the cleanliness of their patients' bathrooms, the accuracy of laboratory tests, and the responsiveness of the nursing staffs when a patient needs a bedpan or a pain medication. For some hospital leaders, this approach will mean a fundamental change of attitude. It will require getting to know their hospital much better. I hope that they are up to the challenge. I also hope that future hospital leaders understand the importance of knowing their departments as they become vice presidents and still remember the importance of knowing their hospital intimately should they become CEOs.

CHAPTER SEVEN

Watch the Dollars

HOSPITALS WASTE tremendous amounts of money. While some say reimbursement systems rewarding sloppy performance are to blame, I think inattentive leadership is to blame.

Responsibility for the financial health of the hospital begins with its leadership. The CEO and senior management are ultimately responsible for the profitability and the strength of the hospital's balance sheet. Under the old cost-based reimbursement systems little attention was paid to the details of hospital financial operations. The "not-for-profit" status was taken far too literally. At long last, all that is changing because of prospective pricing systems and intense competition for patients.

Early warning signals

There are leading indicators that can accurately project problems in the financial operation of a hospital. Some are self-evident; others are more subtle. Both are indicative of the wasteful attitude of management and employees.

Just as there are seven early warning signs for cancer, there are also seven early warning signs for "financial illness.'' Early detection is essential. If we define financial illness as uncontrolled growth of expenses or a general decline in organization health brought about by multiple system failures, then the following warning signs are pertinent:

1. *Unprofitability*—This is the obvious one. It is equivalent to a metastatic disease in that there is a general failure of multiple systems that can ultimately end an organization's life. This is also known as bankruptcy. When a hospital experiences a series of unprofitable years, it is clear it has major underlying financial problems. When operating losses exceed 1 percent of gross income for several years, it indicates a lack of leadership and the inability to either increase revenues or reduce expenses.

2. *Working Capital Erosion*—This is like anemia. When working capital begins to erode, the hospital's future ability to service its financial obligations is threatened. Working capital erosion happens as a consequence of unprofitable operations. There are other causes as well, such as increases in accounts receivable and decreases in accounts payable. Working capital changes should be observed closely by the hospital leadership. Erosion should be avoided if the organization wishes to remain strong and have the necessary resources to expand its facilities in the future.

3. *Capital Replacement*—Hospitals are, of course, capital intensive environments. When things get rough financially, some hospitals begin to cut back on equipment acquisitions. It is the organization equivalent to prolonged loss of physical fitness. When annual new equipment and plant purchases

begin to fall below depreciation expense levels, trouble is sure to follow. To remain competitive, and upgrade equipment and facilities, it is necessary to acquire new equipment at least at the rate of annual depreciation. When acquisitions fall below this level, hospitals are not replacing equipment and facilities at the rate they are becoming obsolete. Physicians and the community notice this. The outcome can be the loss of skilled physicians and ultimately the loss of patients to more progressive facilities.

4. *Accounts Receivable Deterioration*—There is tremendous variance in the abilities of hospitals to collect the money due to them. A sure sign of impending problems is the erosion of accounts receivables. Like excessive unplanned weight loss, it reduces organization energy levels and the ability to "fight off" other diseases. As third party payors become more and more pressed for resources, their strategies have been to slow down payments to hospitals. This puts increasing pressure on hospitals to be efficient in their collections process. The good old-fashioned squeaky wheel mentality has no substitute when it comes to managing accounts receivables. Hospitals that deal aggressively with third party payors get better service and faster turnaround on their receivables. When receivables begin to go up, it is a sure sign of problems to come in other areas.

5. *Accounts Payable Increases*—When hospitals are pressed for cash, one of the first areas of compromise is paying their bills on time. This gets noticed virtually immediately by vendors. When the problems

become serious, vendors may threaten to reduce or discontinue services. In the worst case, they may take more drastic action. More than one hospital has been forced into "Chapter 11" by their vendors. When this takes place, it is usually the culmination of months or sometimes years of frustration. When accounts payable begin to rise, trouble is sure to follow.

6. *Personnel Increases*—Middle managers can increase personnel expenses many ways without adding staff. Thesc arc symptoms of underlying control issues, which can become serious if left unchecked. When overtime and sick time use begins to increase for no apparent reason, productivity deteriorates. This is the organization equivalent to low blood sugar. Part-time workers used beyond their authorized levels cause a deterioration in productivity. Using "temporaries" that do not add to the payroll directly but still cost money is another symptom of impending problems. Lack of control over personnel expenses can lead to the wasting of precious financial resources.

7. *Attention to Detail*—This is the organization equivalent to a leaking aneurism slowly causing death through loss of blood. Many subtle indicators suggest that the leadership is not aware of the hundreds of areas leading to waste. Not taking cash discounts on supply purchases because of cash shortages is a good example. The uncontrolled use of copying machines is another example. Over-using expensive systems like beeper pagers is another symptom. One Chicago hospital even issued its internal auditor a

beeper! Other subtle indicators: the over-dependence on disposables, the increase of service contracts, and other symptoms of organizational laziness that can significantly affect financial performance. They all add up to the same thing, wasted dollars.

Financial leadership test

Hospital leaders need to ask themselves certain key questions continually to ensure the financial well-being of their organizations. The "financial leadership checklist" should be administered at least twice a year to CEOs, assistant administrators, and department managers. If affirmative answers are given to three or more of these questions, the hospital is in trouble.

Financial leadership checklist

___ Are you using disposable cups, plates, and dinnerware to serve meals to your patients (excluding isolation patients)?

___ Are you using outside contract service to manage your housekeeping, laundry, or engineering service?

___ Are you using an outside contract service to manage your physical medicine or pharmacy service?

___ Are you failing to obtain competitive bids for all supply items costing in excess of $1,000 per year?

___ Do you allow physicians to make supply decisions without reference to costs?

___ Do you use disposable water pitchers?

___ Does your total personnel sick time usage exceed 2 percent of worked hours?

___ Does the Board of Directors participate in routine financial decisions?

___ Does the CEO fail to participate in major equipment negotiations?

___ Has your director of purchasing failed to take a vacation in the past 24 months?

These are not facetious questions. There is far too little involvement by the CEO and senior management in purchasing and staffing decisions in hospitals. We are relying too much on outside contract services and lower level supervisors to provide services.

Financial leadership

An organization that is healthy financially is so because of sound financial leadership. Financial leadership means establishing financial values that hold senior management and middle management accountable. Four key financial values will serve any hospital well. If they are incorporated into the leadership style of the organization, excellent financial results can follow. The values are:

1. *Stay Alert*—Hospital leadership should stay continuously alert to the early warning signals of impending financial distress and act quickly when they occur.

2. *Do It Yourself*—Too many hospitals today are relying on outside contractors to do their work for them. This is a symptom of laziness. Hospitals whose average census exceeds 50 patients should be able to find a good housekeeper to keep their hospital clean

without hiring an international conglomerate to do it for them. The phenomenal growth of service and management contract services for hospitals is a poor reflection on hospital leadership. In hospitals that exceed 50 beds there should be a high enough quality leadership to do most if not all services in-house.

3. *Purchase Aggressively*—Old-fashioned competitive bidding and aggressive purchasing practices have no substitute. Using group purchasing arrangements can be helpful, but it should never be substituted for competitive bidding to verify that the "group" prices are the best. Keep in mind that sometimes major vendors penalize group purchasing arrangements because there are marginal hospitals in the group with poor accounts payable practices. Sometimes, even a small hospital with a good track record of paying its bills on time can obtain better prices than a group if it negotiates separately.
4. *People Decisions*—Hospitals have historically not done too well in their people decisions. We should not be adding staffing until growth and activity levels absolutely demand it. We should also be watching sick time and overtime usage much more closely than we have in the past. The old adage that we should not be adding staffing until they "start dropping from exhaustion" could do a great deal to increase productivity in some marginal hospitals.

Some final thoughts

This is not a book about hospital finance. However, the values discussed here and throughout the book suggest that the hospital leadership should become more interested and involved in the financial aspects of their organizations. Money wasted through poor leadership is money not available for taking care of sick people. Hospitals successful in managing their finances are going to be the ones in the future to provide the highest level of service and quality because they won't be wasting precious financial resources.

CHAPTER EIGHT

The Economics of Quality

NAME CALLING, posturing, and behind the scenes maneuvering seem as much at home in a modern health care organization as they do in an emerging third world nation. If we had a nickel for each time a physician accused a CEO or assistant administrator of "practicing medicine" or a CEO accused a physician of "meddling in management," we would be rich indeed.

Is conflict an inevitable part of physician/hospital relationships? Until recently, members of either group would probably have responded with an emphatic "yes." Physician/hospital "turfism" has been accepted as a necessary evil. However, under the new regulatory environment, the answer to this question, at least in successful institutions, will be "no." The economics of quality will draw us together.

To increase quality of care in the future, hospitals must either spend fixed resources more wisely, or increase the resources available externally. While both approaches will result in the same outcome, monies available to enhance patient care quality, many hospitals are jumping too quickly to the latter. They are diversifying into areas well outside their traditional realm of expertise, such as real estate ventures, home care companies, and service corporations. Although this approach is not wrong if implemented successfully, hospitals must not diversify at the expense of their primary mission. Business literature is full of examples of corporate failures and re-trenching that resulted from over-diversification in the 1960s and 1970s. Let us hope hospitals are not headed down that same self-destructive path.

Many zealous hospital leaders overlook opportunities in their own hospitals for financing patient care improvements. All they have to do is apply the basic principles of good management. Given a set of fixed resources, the economics of quality are simply this: to increase quality in one area of a hospital's operation, savings can be made in a different area and reinvested to pay for the improvement. To successfully adopt this approach, the line between hospital leaders "practicing medicine" and physicians "meddling in management" may be less well-defined. We had better be up to the challenge of working together for quality improvements or ultimately our patients could experience the consequences of our failure.

Case of the pacemaker conflict

A hypothetical yet all too common scene is a cardiologist walking down a hospital corridor muttering to himself after leaving the hospital CEO's office. They have just battled over the selection decision for cardiac pacemakers. The cardiologist stuck rigidly to his contention that only the brand of pacemaker that he has been using for the last twenty years is acceptable for patients in "his" hospital. He stuck even more rigidly to his contention that selection of a particular pacemaker configuration for his patients is a purely medical decision, and economics have no place in that decision.

The hospital CEO contended that pacemakers, like any item of medical supplies or equipment, should be subjected to the rigors of competitive bidding. Further, he argued that selection of a pacemaker configuration is both an economic and a medical decision. He cited as an example the cardiologist's practice of always using the most sophisticated and expensive pacemaker configuration for all his patients, even though physicians in other hospitals tailor their pacemaker decision to patient need and life expectancy.

In this unfortunate situation, the cardiologist jumped to the conclusion that the hospital CEO cared little about quality, and presumed that competitive bidding would not be in the best interest of patients. The hospital CEO assumed that the cardiologist's rigidity about pacemaker selection was due more to some special "favors" given him by the pacemaker company than to a real interest in the patient's or hospital's well being. Neither party was right, and the issue of quality care within the context of cost control was lost because of the posturing that inevitably takes place when physicians and hospital leaders disagree.

Times have changed

The primary responsibility for ensuring quality has traditionally rested with physicians. This involved virtually every aspect of operations, including selecting supplies, equipment, and services, and setting employee staffing patterns for the institution. As a result, physicians' day-to-day decisions have had a pervasive influence on hospital operations and on hospital costs. Because the cost impact of their decisions and demands has been of little or no consequence for them, physicians have had no incentive to consider factors other than their patients' immediate well being. But times have changed.

Government has increased hospital regulation, and more recently created a totally new prospective reimbursement system known as Diagnostic Related Groupings (DRGs). Regardless of the lip service paid by government about its intentions, the outcome of its intervention has been to focus on the cost, not on the quality of care. If the focus is to remain foremost on the quality of care, hospitals no longer have the luxury of ignoring costs. Neither do physicians.

Future increases in quality will obviously require money. The question is: Where will the money come from? Opportunities to save money in hospitals are tremendous, especially if physicians and hospital leaders work as a team. Under fixed payment systems, physicians and hospital leaders will need to form partnerships based on sound business principles. This may necessitate some learning and adjustments on both sides. If accomplished successfully, it will allow hospitals and physicians to maintain quality despite diminishing resources. Ultimately, the patients will benefit.

Opportunity areas

Hospitals have historically been very ineffective at purchasing goods, services, and equipment. They have not driven a "hard bargain" to get the best possible value for their money. Ineffective hospital leadership is part of the problem. The lack of real physician concern about costs is another. Here are a few examples:

Equipment

Some physicians have a brand bias when it comes to purchasing medical equipment. When considering new cardiac monitoring systems, some physicians prefer the system they trained with to the exclusion of all others. There is also a tendency to ''overpurchase'' equipment capabilities. Hospitals sometimes purchase cardiac monitoring systems that are too sophisticated for the level of care rendered.

Supply Purchases

Supply purchases represent another savings opportunity area. Again, some physicians have brand biases. Surgeons, for example, will sometimes insist on using their ''favorite'' brand of gloves, even though other less costly ones may be perfectly acceptable. There is also a tendency to overpurchase supplies. This is particularly evident in the case of pre-made trays and kits. Even though a physician or nurse might use only a single catheter out of a pre-packaged disposable myelogram tray, some physicians will ''demand'' that tray, even if it means throwing away 75 percent of the tray's contents unused.

Service Delivery

Some physicians have a tendency to demand availability of non-critical services on a 24-hour basis. Is it really necessary to provide ultrasound twenty-four hours a day seven days a week in a 100 bed hospital? Perhaps not, but some hospitals offer this service around the clock because of a few noisy physicians. Some services are provided, particularly on evening and night shifts, solely to accommodate a minority of physicians' personal habits of making rounds late at night. This is draining resources that might be more effectively spent to benefit all patients.

Personnel

Whether we like it or not, the attitudes of hospital workers, particularly nurses, are changing. The health care team demands respect, to be treated with dignity, and to be seen as knowledgeable professionals. Nurses no longer stand at attention when physicians enter into the nursing station. Neither will nurses tolerate being berated in front of patients or their peers. If that happens, they go elsewhere. Then the hospital is saddled with costs associated with turnover, such as recruiting, hiring, and training of new staff. Patient care suffers as new recruits are continually brought in to care for our patients. Frequently the best employees are the least tolerant of being mistreated by physicians or management. The behavior of a few errant physicians or supervisors is enough to drive good employees to another hospital, a terrible price to pay when good employees, particularly nurses, are hard to recruit and retain.

Consequences and opportunities

When physicians are rigid about brands of supplies or equipment, it handicaps the hospital's purchasing effectiveness. When physicians give vendors the idea that only "their" brand is in the running, vendors take advantage by failing to price competitively. Vendors are in business to make a profit. They have used physician bias and physician influence to maximize profits for their businesses by eliminating competition in hospital purchasing. When physicians assert their bias in service delivery decisions and in employee matters, the end result is to disadvantage the hospital.

Most physicians are probably unaware of the full impact this type of involvement has had on hospitals. And it is probably safe to say that this counter-productive behavior stems not so much from a desire to "meddle in management" but from a lack of incentive, time, or information necessary to consider alternatives other than the familiar or easy. Government has now produced the incentive. It is the hospital leadership's responsibility to commit management time, energy, and resources to research available options, provide comprehensive and relevant information, and facilitate the physicians' involvement in key decision-making areas.

Who is responsible for patient care quality? Physicians and management are jointly responsible. Hospitals that succeed in increasing quality under fixed payment systems will be those in which the physicians and management learn to work together to produce savings which are then reinvested to enhance care quality. Here are a few suggestions.

Physicians and hospital leaders can work more effectively

One area is in supply and equipment acquisition. Physicians can best contribute to the effectiveness of purchasing supplies and equipment by defining generic specifications or needs. Instead of saying, "I want Brand A cardiac monitoring equipment," physicians should define specifically what they need in terms of clinical capability. This definition can then be translated into a set of technical and clinical specifications which is utilized by the hospital's purchasing managers to solicit competitive bids.

The most effective role physicians can play in purchasing supplies and equipment is at the beginning and end of the process. In the beginning, they can assist with the development of clinically significant specifications, and in the end, once the selection has been narrowed to only those products or equipment that meet this criteria, physicians can assist with the selection of the best value.

When physicians become involved in personally negotiating and pre-selecting supply and equipment choices, it compromises the hospital's ability to obtain the best prices.

Physicians should remain flexible during the bid and negotiation process and should not, under any circumstances, interact with vendors directly about their personal preferences. Purchasing and negotiating should be left to the hospital management. Physicians do not have the time, interest or experience to give such functions the appropriate degree of attention. On the other hand, without the assistance of physicians, the hospital management cannot possibly insure that their hospital is acquiring the best possible equipment, service, or supply at the most economic price.

Physicians should also be cognizant of the fact that even the appearance of bids and competition between vendors can produce significant savings. There are countless examples of hospitals obtaining competitive bids for the first time for a supply item. The outcome of the process is that the original supplier retains the business but lowers its prices considerably simply because the supplier did not want to lose the business. The x-ray film business is an excellent example. Many hospitals are saving significant money by initiating a system of bidding on x-ray film now that European and Japanese products are challenging Kodak and Dupont.

Physicians need to recognize the implications of their demands regarding service availability. Is it really necessary to have a pharmacist on duty twenty-four hours a day in a 200 bed hospital, or can nursing supervisors fill the prescriptions on an emergency basis as needed at night? Expectations must be tailored to what can be reasonably afforded. Administrators should communicate with physicians effectively and articulate the economic consequences of service availability charges.

What about employees? The best hospital employees are retained when treated with respect and dignity by the management and physicians. Physicians inclined to berate employees may be those least inclined to change their own behavior. However, they and their physician peers should recognize that the outcome of this behavior may be to drive good employees elsewhere. The hospital may then be saddled with turnover of its best employees. The hospital has a corresponding obligation to ensure that its own management staff functions in a manner promoting retention rather than turnover of its employees. Each time an experienced nurse leaves a hospital, it costs from $4,000 to $6,800 to recruit and train a replacement. Money spent on recruiting and training is then not available for use elsewhere in the hospital's operation.

Outcome of a physician/management partnership

In the worst case, an effective partnership between hospital leaders and physicians will enable a hospital to maintain its quality position in a period of declining or fixed reimbursement. In an optimal situation, it will mean that a hospital has more financial resources to be used for increasing the quality of care.

Surviving without carefully managing costs is impossible. Managing costs is impossible without an effective partnership between medical staff and management. Physicians need a successful hospital, and hospitals need successful physicians. This means that physicians and hospital leaders must change their old confrontational habits. The goal of this partnership is to do a better job for patients. This will be harder to do in the future because of financial and regulatory restrictions on hospitals. But it is increasingly necessary and must become a major priority of medical and administrative staffs.

Pacemakers revisited

Getting back to the pacemaker example. What could have happened differently? If the cardiologist had worked with the hospital to develop a set of clinically sound generic specifications for pacemakers, rather than sticking rigidly to "his" brand, all parties involved might have benefited. A generic set of specifications enables the hospital to consider all pacemaker options meeting the physician-defined criteria and then negotiate the best price.

It is safe to say that when competition is introduced, hospitals are able to negotiate substantially better prices. Had the cardiologist developed the specifications, and then assisted the hospital in making a purchase selection after all the negotiations took place, it is virtually assured the hospital would have achieved savings.

The savings from that negotiation could then have been reinvested into areas that would have benefited the cardiologist's patients. For example, if $20,000 a year was saved, the hospital could have used that savings to add an additional registered nurse in the cardiac care unit to increase the nurse to patient ratio. The cardiologist could certainly view this as a positive outcome, recognizing that his or her input is essential to produce that outcome.

What happens when physicians and hospital leaders form an economic partnership? Resources are expended more effectively and patients benefit from the reinvestment of savings into initiatives that produce a higher quality of care. In other words, we enhance patient care. That is what we all should be working for.

CHAPTER NINE

Hurry Up and Wait

SOME HOSPITAL departments run more for the convenience of the physicians and staff than they do for their customers, the patients. I once asked a hospital dietician why she was serving her patients the evening meal at 4:30 p.m. She said it was important to her staff that they be home by 6 p.m., so patient meal schedules were arranged accordingly. The sad thing is that the dietician saw nothing wrong with that approach, even though she would not think of eating her own evening meal at 4:30 p.m.

Hospital leaders need to take a fresh look at the scheduling and provision of services in their departments. This is where assistant administrators and vice presidents can have a major impact on improving the services for patients in their respective departments. They should begin by putting themselves in the shoes of their customers. They can do this by listening and gathering responses on how well or how poorly the scheduling and delivery of services meets the needs of their customers.

Ancillary service scheduling

The provision of ancillary diagnostic services like laboratory and x-ray exams is a major source of revenue for hospitals. Individual departments schedule patients for their own convenience. For example, when a patient needs an x-ray, the patient or physician usually calls the hospital and makes an appointment. If the procedure requires special preparation like fasting, the department usually issues those instructions. When only one test or procedure is scheduled involving one department, hospitals usually do a reasonable job. When multiple tests and departments are involved, we sometimes fail to keep our patient's needs firmly in mind.

How many times have we heard patients complain that they visited the laboratory first to have blood drawn, only to be kept waiting 90 minutes in radiology? To make matters worse, sometimes the preparations for the lab tests contradict preparations for x-ray procedures, with no one bothering to tell the patient. These scheduling anomalies cause frustration and rescheduled exams and leave patients with the impression that we either do not care or are incapable of coordinating our services.

One California community hospital developed a creative approach to dealing with the scheduling issue. Rather than have patients or physicians call the departments to schedule exams, one central scheduling department handles all ancillary department scheduling. The department is not staffed with clerks, it is staffed with medical professionals knowledgeable in the preparations for all of the clinical exams performed in that hospital. The scheduling department draws on the expertise of ancillary department personnel and upon physicians when necessary. When presented with a request from a physician or patient for a series of diagnostic procedures, the scheduling department sequences the procedures and issues the necessary patient instructions so they are prepared for each department that they visit. When there are contradictions, the department takes the initiative to schedule conflicting procedures on different days and arranges the visit to the hospital around the patient's schedule.

This hospital goes one step further. It provides assistance and a central call-back number for patients so that conflicts and schedule changes are handled through one central scheduling department, rather than a series of departments. When the hospital implemented this program several years ago it achieved an unexpected benefit. It increased productivity. Its ancillary departments scheduled more patients than were previously possible because many of the rescheduled exams caused by poor communication were eliminated.

Each hospital handles scheduling issues its own way. However, it is possible when the leadership takes a firm interest in setting up schedules from the patient standpoint for both patient satisfaction and the efficiency of the ancillary departments to be greatly enhanced.

Surgery scheduling

There have probably been more hospital/physician fights over how to schedule surgery suites than any other single issue, with the possible exception of the size and location of physician parking lots.

The creativity of surgeons to "beat the system" far exceeds the ability of most hospital leaders to create efficient operating room schedules. This, coupled with a propensity on the part of surgeons to want to have their patients prepped and in the operating room two hours before they arrive in the building, causes severe scheduling problems for surgery patients.

Hospitals and physicians must learn to cooperate better when it comes to the scheduling of surgery patients. As hospitals move more toward outpatient surgery, this becomes even more critical. Nothing is more distressful for patients who are scheduled for the "convenience" of day surgery than to arrive two hours before the surgeon is even in the building and to be kept waiting needlessly so the surgeon can begin the case when his schedule permits.

The essential factor in improving the scheduling systems for surgery patients is trust. Hospitals must learn to trust surgeons more and fight less when it comes to scheduling anomalies. If a surgeon or hospital assistant administrator was kept NPO for 12 hours so that a case could begin at 8 o'clock, and then has the case moved to 11 o'clock because of a lab delay, they perhaps might appreciate scheduling problems from a patient's point of view.

Another element in improving surgery schedule from a patient's point of view is coordination. For inpatient surgery, hospitals should do the necessary pre-surgery diagnostic procedures the night before so that all clinical information is ready and waiting for the surgeon. There should be no scrambling around on the day of surgery looking for EKG's and the results of laboratory or radiology exams. For outpatient surgery, hospitals should have STAT capabilities so that necessary procedures can be done quickly and efficiently on the day of surgery, if not several days before. If hospital ancillary departments and physicians' offices could learn to work better together, the outcome would be much more efficient scheduling and much higher satisfaction among their patients.

Why do we wake them?

Hospitals are supposed to be places where sick people come to get better. Then why do some hospitals wake patients up at 4 a.m. to weigh them and take their blood pressure? Why, mostly because of tradition and habit. I know of one midwestern hospital that has a policy of weighing its patients between 4 a.m. and 5 a.m. because a few of the internists make rounds at that time every day, and they insist on having the daily weights on the chart when they arrive. How ridiculous it is to wake a soundly sleeping patient to weigh him or her just because of a physician's early rising habits. Moreover, night shifts usually have the least staffing available to perform such tasks. Although this may sound like an extreme example, there are many examples of inconveniencing patients simply because of tradition.

No one would deny that it is necessary to continuously take vital signs for patients who are critically ill. Hospitals, however, are really not advancing the cause of recovery by taking pulses and blood pressures of most of our patients throughout the night. And how about medication administration schedules? We sometimes pay little if no attention to a patient's rest needs when we order medication on an every-four-hour or every-six-hour schedule. Of course, certain medications have to be given on a rigid schedule. However, there is sometimes little common sense exercised in carrying out these medication schedules.

It is the job of hospital leaders, nursing management in particular, to take a more active role in deciding upon patient routines. Head nurses are in an excellent position to assist physicians with making reasonable schedule judgements. They will need backing from middle and top management when scheduling changes affect physician traditions. However, if patient needs are kept firmly in mind, reasonable accommodations can be reached with both groups.

Common courtesy

Regardless of how efficient or how customer-oriented a hospital is, tests or services will sometimes be delayed. When that is the case, effective hospitals have mechanisms in place to communicate with the customers. For example, when the ultrasound machine breaks down in x-ray and a morning's worth of patients are going to be cancelled, a call-back mechanism should be implemented immediately so that those patients are notified and rescheduled at their convenience. Nothing is worse to a patient than arriving promptly for a 10 a.m. ultrasound only to find out that the machine broke down the night before. Nothing the technician says at that moment is going to make up for the hassle that patient had in arranging for a babysitter and scheduling time off from work to arrive at the hospital on time. Another important consideration is keeping people informed if inevitable delays occur while they are waiting. If an exam is going to be delayed for an hour and the patient is already present, a representative of the department should check back with the patient every 30 minutes or so and let them know the status. If a patient is unable to wait, a follow-up appointment should be scheduled on the spot at the patient's convenience, rather than the department's.

Communication and courtesy are the keys. One progressive Illinois hospital makes it a point to call all of its outpatients the evening before scheduled laboratory, x-ray, and EKG exams to confirm the appointments and to check whether or not the patients have understood the necessary preparations for their individual procedure. That hospital truly understands that good communication leads to effective scheduling. They also go one step further and call patients the day after an exam to be sure that there have been no untoward effects or follow-up questions that are bothering the patients. This hospital was able to provide these services without adding any staff because they discovered that there were so many fewer cancelled exams through better communication that staff time was freed up to make the necessary pre- and post-exam courtesy calls.

Scheduling is a leadership issue

Hospitals have been able to get away with inefficient scheduling and poor attention to customer needs for years. Now, with increased competition, enlightened hospitals are taking scheduling, communication, and common courtesy seriously. This, of course, greatly benefits the customer.

Understand that scheduling is a leadership issue, not simply a systems issue. Arranging patient communication and scheduling to meet customer needs rather than department or staffing needs recognizes that we are in business to serve customers. The dietary department is not in business to do anything but serve meals to patients on their schedules, not the dietary department schedule. We should be scheduling ancillary, diagnostic, and therapeutic services around patient needs rather than around staff and physician needs. To accomplish this, assistant administrators and department heads must understand the importance of customer needs. They need to be held accountable by their CEOs for arranging services along customer lines rather than departmental lines. There are a few shining examples of hospitals who have understood and acted upon those customer needs. The rest of us should emulate those hospitals as quickly as possible.

CHAPTER TEN

The Challenge of Teamwork

MORE THAN EVER, there is a crying need for hospital leaders to foster teamwork among management, employees and physicians. The importance of teamwork becomes more critical as the reimbursement strategies for hospitals are changing. Under the old cost-based systems, the more tests and procedures which were performed and the longer patients stayed, the more money hospitals made. Now, under prospective reimbursement systems, the opposite is true. The changes taking place in medicine today call for shorter lengths of stay, more focus on outpatient services and less use of ancillary tests.

These changes are having profound effects on patients. As patient stays become shorter, anxiety over discharge grows higher. Patient anxiety is much influenced by the attitudes of employees and physicians who care for those patients. One cop-out option is for hospitals and physicians to "blame" the system. This does not help patients. Although some of the system changes are beyond our control, we must learn not only to cope with them, but to continue providing high-quality services under the new constraints. This requires a thorough understanding of the new reimbursement systems by all parties and a concerted effort to work within them while providing the necessary quality desired by our customers.

The first step

The first step in developing more effective teamwork under the reimbursement systems is education. Hospital leaders must educate their physicians and rank and file employees to understand the new prospective payment systems. They must also help them understand the pre-admission screening systems and assigned length of stay programs which are being undertaken by many third party payors. These systems create great frustration among patients and it is necessary for employees and physicians to understand these pressures and respond to patient questions about them.

When educating staffs, concentrate on admitting personnel, nursing staff, business office staff, and physicians. These are the individuals who will most likely receive the brunt of the frustrations and the most questions from patients. It is important that they articulate consistent responses to frustrated patients. In other words, when a Medicare patient has questions about the DRG system, the admitting clerk should be able to answer them. The nursing staff should also have enough of a working knowledge of DRGs to help the patient understand how the system works.

The discharge dilemma

Patients are indeed going home sooner than they did in years past. This is partly the result of advances in medicine, which make shorter stays possible. Only a few years ago hospitals were keeping cataract patients for a week with sand bags around their head so that they could not move. Now hospitals perform the same surgery and send patients home in a matter of hours with no untoward effects.

Changes in the reimbursement system are also causing decreased lengths of stay for Medicare patients and for other patients covered by third party insurance. These patients are going home sicker than they did in years past. Although that does not necessarily mean that bad outcomes will follow, hospitals need to ensure that a patient is not discharged if the patient's condition warrants continued stay. This is where hospital leaders need to take a firm stand. The hospital CEO and senior management should let their medical staff know that, regardless of the reimbursement implications, patients must not be discharged if it is medically contraindicated. Physicians should have these assurances from the hospital leadership. Patients deserve it. To do otherwise sacrifices quality and invites litigation from dissatisfied patients.

Also make sure that there is a coordinated effort ensuring discharged patients receive optimal follow-up and home services if they need them. Excellent home care services and other support services which can assist discharged patients are available in most communities. It is the job of the hospital leadership to marshal these services whenever necessary to assist discharged patients. The utilization of home care, patient transportation services, meals on wheels, hospice services, and so on needs to be coordinated to the best possible advantage of discharged patients. Many hospitals utilize their social services departments or discharge planners to ensure that this coordination takes place. It is certainly not necessary that hospitals provide each of these community services directly, but it is necessary that they are aware of the services and coordinate with them so that discharged patients receive the appropriate care.

Attitudes make all the difference

The attitudes of the staff and physicians who come in contact with patients make a tremendous difference on the attitudes of patients upon discharge. Nothing could be worse than a nurse responding inappropriately to a patient or a family member who is concerned about discharge. Nurses skilled in appropriate responses can do much to ease the anxiety of patients and family members when it is time for a patient to return home. These counseling skills should be taught by physicians and hospital leaders.

Staff members who come in contact with patients should receive some training in identifying and referring problems appropriately. For example, it is just as important for the housekeeper to recognize the signs of high anxiety as it is for the nurse. It may not be possible for the housekeeper to provide financial counseling, but he or she certainly should be trained to refer those problems to a member of the nursing staff who can then take appropriate action. In this way, all hospital staff members are working as a team to identify and resolve patient problems.

Another approach to ensuring that patients are appropriately coping with discharges are follow-up phone calls. A Massachusetts hospital pioneered follow-up phone calls to all discharged patients to determine if the appropriate follow-up systems are in place, such as home care and meals on wheels. These calls give the hospital an opportunity to form an excellent "last impression" in the patient's mind. They also occasionally identify significant problems, which can then be referred to the appropriate hospital services for resolution.

Bringing it all together

A Wisconsin community hospital has formulated an excellent approach demonstrating the power of teamwork in a community hospital setting. A prototype physician and staff "vascular team" was conceived by the hospital's vascular surgeon. The team included a surgeon, operating room nurses, intensive care unit nurses, and a head nurse.

The vascular team was assembled to improve communication and the quality of care for patients undergoing vascular surgery. The accomplishments of this team were dramatic and demonstrate what is possible when a coordinated physician, staff, and management effort is developed. The team began meeting "before work" once a week to consider the problems of its vacular surgery patients. It created a completely new approach in dealing and communicating with patients, and along the way even began saving the hospital some money.

The first move by the vascular team was to implement pre- and post-operative visits for the patient and family. The surgeon and operating room nurses visit the patients prior to the surgery to explain the surgical procedures, risks, and the post-operative course. These are not the typical two-minute "consent" discussions. They are high quality counseling sessions that give the patient and family members sufficient time with the professionals to ask all the questions on their minds. This team also visits the patient post-operatively and consults with family members again, giving them the opportunity to ask any questions that have arisen as a result of the surgery.

The team also began carefully examining the various procedures and protocols used during vascular surgery cases and the costs of various supply items utilized during the operation. Now physicians and nurses examine bills item by item to see if there is an opportunity to reduce patient costs. As a result of these examinations, a number of changes were made that had no ill effects on the quality of surgery cases, but did effectively reduce costs. For example: disposable gowns were eliminated in favor of reusable ones; sutures were left unopened until needed, eliminating waste; and several catheters were re-evaluated and substitutes made, reducing costs while maintaining the quality of the surgical care.

Perhaps the most significant contribution of the vascular team is the preparation for a patient's discharge and subsequent follow-up. A series of patient instructions were assembled and an excellent discharge packet put together for the family members and the patient to ensure that follow-up instructions were followed. The team even designed a call-back card with key phone numbers and a diagram of the patient's surgery. A copy of this card appears in Figure 5.

The call-back card gives the patient and family members easy-to-follow instructions for follow-up if untoward events or questions occur after discharge. The team's experience with this approach suggests that not many calls are received; however, there is a much higher level of patient comfort knowing that questions can and will be followed-up quickly when they do arise.

The vascular team concept is being expanded in the Wisconsin hospital to cover other types of cases, like orthopedic and obstetrical cases. It has proven that a multi-disciplinary team of physicians, nurses, and management can

FIGURE 5

VASCULAR PATIENT INFORMATION CARD

Beloit Memorial Hospital

Vascular Laboratory

Mon. - Fri. 8:00-4:30 364-5127

Please call if you have any questions or problems

After 4:30 call;

Answering Service	365-1214
John Roehl (home)	362-8454
Dr. Katz (home)	365-9037

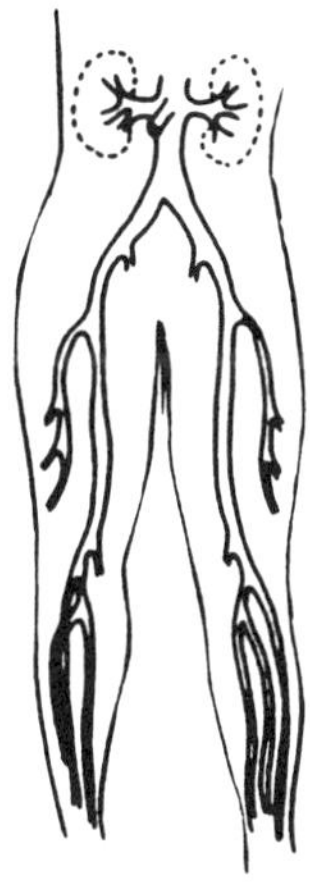

Operation ____________________

____

____

Date ____________________

improve the level of communication, reduce hospital costs, and ease anxieties at the time of discharge through specific discharge instructions and follow-up mechanisms.

Lessons of the vascular team

Patients are going home sooner now, and more outpatient work is being done because of changes in the reimbursement methodologies. These changes are here to stay, and how we respond to them is a measure of our leadership capabilities. If hospitals send patients home in a state of high anxiety following shorter hospital stays, it is a poor reflection of their leadership. If they perform outpatient procedures without the necessary preparation and follow-up, the stage is set for bad medical and social outcomes. At the same time, hospital exposure to litigation is increased.

It is possible, and indeed necessary, for hospitals to use a teamwork approach with their employees and physicians to cope with the changes wrought by new directions in hospital reimbursement. We can shorten hospital stays and perform more outpatient procedures if we have the appropriate coordination mechanisms in place. The vascular team example gives a glimpse of how powerful a coordinated effort can be. Let it be a challenge to all hospitals to formulate their own approaches that maintain or enhance quality and reduce patient stays and associated health care expenditures.

CHAPTER ELEVEN

Marketing Starts at the Top

MARKETING is a "hot" buzzword in the healthcare business. It is seen by some as the solution to all of our problems, the magic elixir which will bring hospitals back from the brink of mediocrity.

There is too much marketing puffery and not enough marketing leadership in hospitals today. The growth of staff positions such as "vice president of marketing" is diagnostic. Ten years ago, whoever heard of a vice president of marketing in a hospital? It is estimated that more than 2000 hospitals have one or more senior staff executives in a marketing position. One of the quickest ways to give a hospital CEO an inferiority complex is to make fun of him because he does not employ a vice president of marketing. The rush into marketing is part trendiness and part substance. Unfortunately, many hospital leaders are getting into marketing more as a function of following a fad than as a well thought-out strategy. Perhaps they never heard Peter Drucker explain that "marketing is what makes selling unnecessary."

Hospital leaders can learn many marketing lessons from business. Lee Iacocca, for example, has taught us that marketing is more a function of identifying products that the marketplace desires, like the mini-vans, than merely sales hype.

What the public did not realize was that the successful mini-van creation was based not on an intuitive flash of brilliance by Iacocca, but on careful market research. The research identified a segment of the car buying population wanting a vehicle roomier than a conventional car, but not as big as the vans that were available in the early 1980s.

Marketing is not a simple concept. It is not something that can be delegated to a staff vice president with positive results to follow immediately. Leadership in marketing, however, is a by-product of good common sense.

Finding out what's happening

The danger some hospital leaders face is assuming they know intuitively what is happening in their marketplaces. They listen to articulate doctors, department heads, and patients. They assimilate all of the information they receive daily and form an impression of what is happening. Sometimes they are right. Many times they are not.

The first serious step in marketing is to objectively understand the marketplace and the customers. Although there are many successful techniques, there is really no substitute for objective community market research. This can be done through focus groups, statistical sampling, or any of the other available techniques used successfully for decades in industry. Market research should be the starting point for any new long-range plan or new service or product development. Hospitals are known for creating "white elephants" by converting intuitive flashes of brilliance into new services without doing any basic research to determine whether anyone wants to buy those services.

A good example of a white elephant creation was a suburban Illinois hospital that wanted to create an industrial medicine center several years ago. An articulate physician was able to convince the hospital board to proceed with a first-class program for executive physicals. A delegation from the hospital even visited Japan to study their methods. After spending a considerable amount in start-up expenses, the new program was launched. It was an immediate failure because it did not attract any customers. The hospital then hired a vice president of marketing to "sell" the program, and still it failed to attract customers.

Finally, the hospital hired a few part-time nurses to contact businesses to find out why they were not buying. The insights from this customer "research" led to renaming, repricing, and reconfiguring the service to meet customer needs. Then, and only then, did the program succeed. If only they had started with customer research first they might have saved hundreds of thousands of dollars, not to mention the frustrations of the program creators.

Another starting point in assessing hospital marketplace is to determine user satisfaction. This does not mean handing out "comment cards" upon discharge. Only a small percentage of cards are ever returned. There was a time when this type of feedback was helpful. It allowed hospitals to focus on problems. But currently there is a much stronger need to get a more careful assessment of both problem areas and strength areas to ensure we are being responsive to our customers.

To accomplish this, hospitals should create statistically significant samples of their customers and then thoroughly question them about the hospital's services. There is no substitute for direct customer feedback, although it is not very much in vogue among today's hospital leaders. Although often delegated to subordinates, talking face to face with several customers each and every day is one way to keep a leader in tune with how the folks that are buying our services respond to them. It can be a humbling experience, as well as a terribly rewarding experience, depending on how well hospitals are satisfying their customers.

Assessing physician satisfacation is another major concern. However, some hospital leaders may appropriately point out that most physicians are never satisfied. Nevertheless, hospital leaders should determine what our physician needs are and meet those needs as best they can.

Marketing begins with an assessment. This assessment is a continuous process and should involve talking with customers, physicians, and community. Do not fall into the trap of believing every noisy physician or patient speaks for the whole group. This is seldom the case. The only way to find out what customers think is to objectively measure their perceptions through market research techniques.

When surveying the community it is a good idea to administer the same questionnaire to hospital employees. Employees can be leading indicators of what the community thinks. For example, if the quality of a hospital is declining, the employees know this well before the community does. They also know about improvements before the community. Employee perceptions about the quality of their own facility are very important to hospital leaders, particularly if they are trying to improve the hospital's reputation. They must first convince employees that improvements are indeed being made. Only then can they hope to convince the community. An Illinois community hospital learned that lesson the hard way when its community market research determined that its own nurses were telling their friends and neighbors not to use their hospital because it was so "understaffed."

Strength and weakness assessment

Identifying strengths and weaknesses is a very important part of marketing. All hospitals have some services that are better than others. Though difficult to admit, it is just not possible to have every single service and every single department achieving at the highest possible levels at the same time. It has been said many times that the worst thing you can do with a mediocre product or service is to promote it. For hospitals, this applies at least as much, if not more, than in industry. The worst thing you can do with a poor emergency room service is advertise. More people will use it and become disenchanted. On the other hand, if a hospital has a particularly good rehabilitation department, they should do everything in their power to promote it.

Identifying the strengths and weaknesses of our hospitals is a subjective process to some degree, but hospital leaders should be able to do it effectively by reviewing patient outcomes and evaluating physician and management strengths. If leaders cannot do that, they do not belong in leadership positions. After hospitals have identified their strengths, they can evaluate how those strengths can be used to promote the hospital and to position the hospital effectively in the external environment.

What's out there?

It is up to hospital leaders to determine what their competition is. Market research can help in this regard, and so can common sense. Evaluating competing hospitals is an important part of the marketing process. Hospitals should know what their competitors' strengths and weaknesses are. Doing market research in a competitor's service area is one way to determine this. Keeping well-informed about competitive hospital activities through newspaper clipping reviews and other common sense approaches is also quite important. Hospitals should assess what competitive threats exist in their marketplace. Who's developing new HMOs and PPOs? Who's likely to put together an ''Emergi-'' or ''Surgi-Center''? What other physician clinics are looking hard at our service area and what are they likely to try next?

A small dose of paranoia seems to be present in many good leaders. Assuming your competitors are ''out to get you'' can be a healthy attitude for hospital leaders if not taken to the extreme. Watching for weaknesses and opportunities to utilize your own hospital strengths is part of the marketing process, and without question the ultimate responsibility of the leader.

Integrating marketing and operations

Resources and energy should be channelled into developing the hospital's strengths and resolving its problems. Building on strengths and reducing at least the glaring problems is a prerequisite to promoting any hospital. It is a terrible thing for a hospital to refer to itself as ''world class,'' ''the best,'' or any other such ridiculous label when it cannot get hot food to the patients, or when it has surly nurses that barely speak civilly to patients. Good words of advice are to ''get thy house in order'' before entering the magic world of marketing and promotion.

Building a committed physician and management group is also essential in developing a marketing-oriented organization. It does little or no good if the leaders are on board and the employees delivering the services are on another planet. It does no good if the management and employees are on board and the physicians are marching to a different drummer. On the other hand, a leadership group who can get their managers, employees, and physicians all moving in the same direction has an unstoppable force behind them.

The physician as marketer

Market research has taught hospitals that physicians can be powerful marketers. I do not necessarily mean putting them on TV smiling at a two-year-old. I mean arranging for them to be seen in the community. Having a radiologist talk to a group of senior citizen women about the new mammography unit is a great way to advertise, better than newspaper ads. Having obstetricians talk to young women's groups about the birthing center is great advertising too. Look for ways to get positive exposure for your physicians. It will build their practices and contribute to your hospital's services because you will be known as a hospital whose physicians are anxious to speak to community groups. Word of mouth has proven time and time again that it's the most powerful referral mechanism for physicians.

Hospital leaders should give their physicians a helping hand to make the best use of their time. Take care of nonmedical details for them, like scheduling and preparing the audiovisuals. Hospitals will be rewarded with the most powerful advertising of all–word of mouth. Most physicians are not anxious to take up valuable time promoting hospitals, so the leaders will have to be persuasive. If successful, they will be harnessing a powerful marketing force for their hospital and medical staff.

Some thoughts about advertising

There are as many different advertising concepts as there are firms. At best, however, advertising is a questionable enterprise for hospitals. There is little evidence to confirm that hospital advertising influences the marketplace in any substantial way. Many communities, both large and small, can attest that spending large sums of money on hospital advertising has not really influenced hospital selection very much. It was rumored, for example, that hospitals and HMOs in a large midwest community spent over $1 million in a recent 12-month period on advertising with no change at all in relative market share at the end of the ad series.

But common sense and keeping up with competition is forcing many CEOs to concede hospital advertising is here to stay. Hospital leaders must be open-minded and progressive about its presence and value. Common sense should be the guide in selecting the various advertising vehicles, which can range from television and radio to newspapers, magazines, direct mail, and word of mouth.

One of the most effective things hospital leaders can do in preparing an advertising program is to show it to the hospital's constituent groups before it is launched. This includes physicians, employees, management, and maybe even the hospital volunteers. No matter what the advertising effort covers, if the various groups in the hospital see it in advance and have an opportunity to understand its genesis, they are much better prepared to support the advertising once it has been released. It is unfortunate, but some hospitals launch major advertising efforts without even showing them to their own physicians and employees. This does nothing but cause resentment and minimize the full positive impact that advertising can have.

The timing of advertising is also important. Being first does not necessarily guarantee success. Superbly designed and eloquently written ads do not guarantee success either. More than one hospital in a blue collar town has published advertisements which only a Ph.D. could understand. When physicians get involved in advertising, they tend to write for themselves, rather than for the customers that they are trying to influence. A good rule of thumb is never let physicians write advertising copy. However, they can be productively engaged in the advertising process by reviewing concepts and overall strategies.

How does one measure advertising effectiveness? I doubt if anyone really knows. Perhaps the effect on hospital image can be measured through market research studies; however, no one has yet been able to establish a real cause and effect relationship between advertising and increased or decreased hospital business. In short, it is safe to say that some advertising is here to stay, and we better increase our level of sophistication if we want to prosper in the future.

Integrating creativity and advertising

Although it was previously stated that advertising alone does not success make, there are many current examples of using advertising to successfully promote well thought out and researched services. Two of the most creative service areas that come to mind are senior citizen services and women's health services.

Ask a senior citizen what worries him or her most about their health, and they will likely answer the fear of catastrophic illness depleting their financial resources and the paperwork associated with Medicare claims and supplemental insurance. A number of progressive hospitals are creating services to deal with both fears. They are establishing billing services specifically tailored to senior citizens and related programs to drop Medicare deductibles and copayments. These programs, coupled with effective advertising programs, have clearly demonstrated that market share can shift favorably in a competitive multi-hospital environment.

Women's health services are another example. Although we have known for years that women select most of the physicians and hospitals for their family, only recently have hospitals and physician groups created special programs aimed at satisfying women's health needs. Many successful programs are now in place stressing the full range of women's health issues, not just obstetrics. These programs, coupled with excellent advertising programs, have also shifted market share in competitive hospital environments.

The essence of marketing

The real essence of marketing is not advertising; it is creating satisifed customers. No matter how beautiful the TV ads, no matter how wonderful the radio jingles, satisfied customers and positive word of mouth are still the best advertising vehicle for a service industry like ours. The best way to advertise any hospital is to produce satisfied customers. These satisfied customers tell their friends and neighbors, their sons and daughters, and their beauticians. Those folks tell other folks, and pretty soon you have a reputation you can be proud of.

No amount of advertising in the world is going to compensate for unsatisfied customers. My advice to hospital leaders is first to know what your customers think. Second, emphasize the strengths in your hospital. Third, do a little advertising to promote those strengths, but keep 90 percent of your marketing efforts focused on the everyday items which satisfy or dissatisfy your customers.

Think of it this way: which would you rather rely on, an advertisement or a personal recommendation from a good friend? Answer that question, and you'll have grasped the essence of hospital marketing.

CHAPTER TWELVE

Planning: The Shorter the Better

IT IS NOT BY ACCIDENT that this is the shortest chapter in this book. The problem with planning in today's hospitals is that there is too much emphasis on planning and not enough emphasis on doing. Planning, especially when carried out by staff assistants, is losing some of its glitter. Many large corporations who led the charge to form strategic planning departments in the 1960s and 1970s are now leading the charge to dismantle them. Corporate giants like General Electric and IBM are dismantling their planning departments and delegating planning back to line management. This is a trend that bears duplicating in the hospital industry.

The consultant trap

Not too long ago, many hospital leaders' idea of planning was to hire an outside consultant who charged a very substantial fee to produce a two-inch thick "strategic plan." This plan would eventually be filed in an inaccessible place, never to see the light of day again after it was duly presented to the hospital board. Another common approach was to delegate planning to a staff planner or planning department.

The results were the same in most cases—an elegant document but little commitment by the line organization to go out and achieve it.

This is an exaggeration, but not too much. Hospital leaders have relied excessively on other people to do their planning for them. Obviously, hospitals have to use outside expertise to do highly technical work like demographic projections, market research, CON investigations, capital financing and evaluations. But they should not have to have consultants tell them what their strengths and weaknesses are and how to best meet the needs of their customers. Peters and Waterman observed in *In Search of Excellence* that "one of the most thoughtful strategic plans we've seen is put together by the president, with the only staff help coming from his secretary and the part-time work of his department and division managers. He had no staff, let alone planning staff." They were referring to the $1 billion Ore-Ida company.[10]

Thousands of planners are employed in hospitals. What do these planners actually produce for patients? A difficult question to answer, unless of course you ask one of these planners. In that case, you can expect a one-inch thick, 200 page report complete with charts and graphs on the subject within a week. Planning, in and of itself, is a process. It does not produce an outcome that helps us take better care of patients. Planners are far removed from the "action" of delivering the service for which hospitals are in business to provide. Additionally, planners usually do not implement anything. Implementation is left to the line managers, who in many cases had little to do with the original plan development. Last, and certainly not least, planners and their staffs cost a lot of money. Outside "strategic planning" consultants cost even more money. It's time hospital leaders asked what is actually being produced for those consulting dollars and whether or not they could do it cheaper and better themselves.

A long-range plan

I would like to suggest a different planning approach. The approach is that the hospital CEO and his senior management, together with key members of the medical staff and board, should be the planners. These key people should have the vision for where a hospital is going. If they are really effective leaders, that vision will be clearer than an outside consultant's or inside planner's interpretation. Hiring some outside expertise to do the demographics, market research, and other technical assignments is fine. But let us keep the real matter of planning among the hospital's leaders, not the staff people or consultants.

It does not take a tremendous amount of effort to produce a good "home-grown" long-range plan. A CEO, several of the key staff members, some physician leaders, and board members can produce an excellent long-range plan in several months. The starting point for the plan should be the creation, or updating, of the hospital mission statement. The essential element for creating a good mission statement is focus. Many mission statements are meaningless puffery. A good mission statement need not be longer than a paragraph or two, and should focus on one or two key aspects of the hospital's purpose. It should also be realistic and doable. "What do we want to be?" is the key question the planners must answer. The mission statement must answer the question clearly and concisely. Once the mission statement is established, the other elements of the plan can proceed.

The next step is a thorough evaluation of the competitive marketplace, community market research information, and a thorough analysis of the hospital's strengths and weaknesses. When that analysis is complete, then the development of assumptions and objectives can begin. Several examples of appropriate long-range plan assumptions and objectives are included in Appendix A. Note that they are strategic rather than operational in nature. Note also that they are measurable.

The time frame for long-range planning is getting shorter and shorter. It's not uncommon to find a long-range plan covering 3-5 years. Not too long ago long-range plans were 10 years or more. Our marketplace is changing much too rapidly for 10-year plans. A small group of committed top executives, physicians and board members can produce an excellent long-range plan. It may not look as sophisticated as the $100,000 "strategic plan" of a major consulting company, but it has a much better chance of being implemented because the leaders doing the implementing are the same leaders that created it.

When completed, the long-range plan should be distributed to all members of management, medical staff, and board members. Additionally, special presentations should be made to all employees and volunteers so they too have a thorough understanding of where the hospital is headed.

Operating plans

Once a long-range plan is finished, it can be used as the basis for short-range (e.g. one year) operating plans. Some hospitals get too carried away with management by objective systems by creating hundreds of individual objectives. First select three to five overall "corporate" objectives for the year. These corporate objectives come from the long-range plan. Then, develop three to five detailed objectives for each department and nursing unit that contribute to accomplishing the corporate objectives. It takes mental discipline to decide what are the three to five most important things to accomplish in a year. Effective leaders possess the ability to focus on the items that will make a difference. Creating hundreds of objectives can lead to many objectives of questionable value.

An important characteristic of a good annual operating plan is that its objectives must be measurable. "Improving productivity," "decreasing turnaround time" and "enhancing morale" are examples of poorly drawn objectives. Examples of tightly drawn departmental objectives are as follows:

- *Personnel Department* Implement systems to ensure a three-week turnaround on filling 95 percent of non-professional vacancies and an eight week turnaround on 90 percent of professional vacancies to be evaluated at the end of each month.
- *Nursing Department Medical/Surgical Unit* Administer pain medication within 10 minutes of the time requested. Once a month the pain medication request log and patients' charts will be monitored for meeting established standards. Additionally, ten patients will be interviewed at random to test compliance each month.
- *Birthing Services Department* Achieve 50 additional obstetrical deliveries in 19__ resulting in an increase in revenue of $100,000.

Reporting and follow-up

Planning is just a process. Even if it is done by line managers, it is still just a process. Planning is only good for moving an organization ahead. Moving ahead means accomplishing what the plan says and reporting back the results. A wise hospital board member once remarked that he expects his hospital CEO and senior executives to "plan the work, and then work the plan." That says it all.

There is no magic answer on how much is too much with reference to reporting, but communicating results at least quarterly with the major constituent groups such as employees, management, physicians, and board members is probably sufficient. There is nothing more sobering for a hospital CEO than having to walk into a board meeting with nothing accomplished during the past quarter. On the other hand, there is nothing so rewarding as being able to report positive progress and accomplishment of those things which you set out to do. That is what leadership is all about.

CHAPTER THIRTEEN

Quality: Whose Job Is It?

WHO IS RESPONSIBLE for dealing with an elderly physician who drifts in and out of reality but still insists on taking care of patients when he is lucid? Who is responsible when a poorly-trained ICU nurse on the night shift does not recognize and promptly report a significant clinical deterioration to the attending physician? What do you do with a laboratory technician who is not astute enough to recognize a seriously abnormal test result and report it immediately to the patient's physician? And who is supposed to watch for the registered nurse addicted to Demerol whose judgement is severely affected when taking care of patients? And whose fault is it if an extremity turniquet used in a hand surgery case squeezes the upper arm too tightly during an operation and damages vital nerves, causing post-surgical motor deficits?

No excuses

These are basic quality issues. Although each issue is different in character, hospital leaders are responsible for avoiding or dealing with these issues as they occur within their institutions. It takes insight and it sometimes takes courage to deal with these problems, but effective leaders do not look for excuses—they look for results.

It is not possible for hospital leaders to observe every medication that is administered, to monitor each x-ray for appropriate exposure, or to observe every physical therapy treatment. It is, however, the job of hospital leaders to make line managers accountable for every transaction in their areas of responsibility. Head nurses must understand that they are responsible for the treatments rendered by their staff. Chief pharmacists must understand that they are responsible for the actions of every single pharmacist and every medication order filled. Chief engineers must understand that they are accountable for the condition of the buildings and each item of equipment within the hospital campus.

Identify quality problems

How can hospital leaders observe and measure the quality of care? Much has been written on the subject of risk management and the measurement of quality. An essential element of any quality accountability system is a mechanism to identify and report aberrations. The incident report is the generic term used to describe a specific problem area or issue. Most incident reports contain areas to explicitly define a problem and any planned follow-up action. Regardless of the format, an incident reporting system is critical in the overall quality accountability system. The question then becomes, "Who reviews the incident reports?" Hospital leaders should review all incident reports that identify harm that has come to a patient, visitor, or staff member.

Defining harm can be difficult. However, if common

sense is applied it becomes easier. If a patient receives incorrect treatment or has blood drawn because of an identification error, consider that to be a form of harm. Admittedly, this is a rather liberal interpretation of harm. In larger institutions, this means hospital leaders will have to review many incident reports. However, if they put themselves in the position of the patient, they would agree having blood drawn needlessly or receiving someone else's x-ray is inflicting harm. Perhaps reviewing these incident reports will motivate hospital leaders to be more aggressive in dealing with quality issues, such as patient identification errors that result in a patient receiving the wrong diet or medication.

Incident reporting systems are valuable in identifying emerging patterns. An upstate New York hospital especially good at identifying patterns once pinpointed a single nursing unit as having an inordinately high number of medication errors. After a thorough review, it was determined that a particularly self-motivated RN had implemented her own policy of medication delivery. That RN was responsible for a great number of medication errors and confusion among her RN peers before her actions were discovered. Pattern reviews can identify many solvable quality problems. For example, one hospital's review of patient falls indicated that a change in the administration schedule for diuretics considerably reduced the number of falls. How? The incident report trend analysis indicated that patients on diuretics were particularly vulnerable to falls while walking to the bathroom soon after receipt of their medication. Revision of the medication schedule made it possible to have more staff available to assist patients in their trips to the bathroom, which significantly reduced the number of falls. Hence, bruises, abrasions, and even a few broken hips were avoided.

Regardless of the system used to identify problems, follow-up on problems is the essential ingredient in obtaining higher quality. No institution is perfect. Mistakes will occur. High quality leaders, however, instill in their staff the importance of follow-up action. Mediocre leaders do not. This accounts for their mediocrity. Follow-up action can take various avenues, such as changing medication schedules and increasing the education programs for identified areas of deficiency. It can also mean the reassignment of staff members who prove themselves unable to fulfill responsibilities. Although it is not frequent, high quality hospitals do not hesitate to reduce a registered nurse to licensed practical nurse status or even nursing assistant status if she can no longer fulfill registered nurse obligations. Also, well-led organizations do not hesitate to let staff members go who consistently prove they are unable to uphold the institution's quality standards.

Many other informative channels are available to the hospital leader in addition to incident reporting systems. One of the best is listening. Listening to the patients can be an enlightening experience and can help identify many quality related issues. Listening to physicians can also identify potential problem areas.

Family members are also a good source of information on quality related matters. Hospital leaders sometimes get defensive when family members complain about the quality of care; however, if they spent less time being defensive and more time listening to what family members have to say they would obtain information that could help improve the hospital's services. The observations of the management staff are also useful in identifying problem areas. Regardless of the source, enlightened leaders take actions to resolve quality related problems and accept the full responsibility for the quality of care in their institution. A reputation for quality, or lack of it, is usually deserved. One need not look any further than the hospital's leaders and their commitment to quality to determine whether or not the hospital practices what it preaches.

What about equipment?

Several years ago, a major manufacturer of hospital beds issued an alert to all hospitals using a particular model electric bed. A little investigation revealed that the reason for the alert was that a pediatric patient had been crushed to death when the bed had malfunctioned. There is a tremendous amount of complex medical equipment in hospitals, ranging in complexity from blood pressure measuring devices to multimillion dollar diagnostic equipment such as MRI Scanners. Who is accountable for ensuring that the equipment does not malfunction and inflict harm? Hospital leaders are accountable.

Of course, it's not possible for hospital leaders to personally inspect each item of equipment in their organization. Therefore, systems must be set up to ensure that equipment is running properly. Preventative maintenance programs are the most important. It is widely known that various accrediting bodies require strict attention to preventive maintenance programs. Hospital leaders rely on their engineering department to perform these tasks. However, the hospital CEO and vice president in charge of engineering should occasionally select an item or two of equipment at random and check personally to see if the preventative maintenance program is actually working as it was intended.

Hospital leaders should never accept the word of a subordinate or fully trust a system when it comes to matters of quality. They should personally make sure that equipment checks are actually being carried out.

Even with the best preventative maintenance program equipment breakdowns and failures are inevitable. Prompt response should follow any equipment malfunction. You have heard the old expression, "The part's on order"? It is uttered thousands of times in hospitals around the country. Telling a grieving mother that the part for a fetal heart monitor that might have saved her newborn was on order will be of little comfort. If hospital leaders had to face a family with that kind of story, they would have less patience with their engineering department and parts manufacturers when it comes to prompt deliveries. To put it bluntly, it is the CEO's and his senior management's responsibility to ensure that equipment is repaired promptly. No excuse is accepted for late deliveries and failure to return equipment to good working order.

Another important aspect to the operation of equipment in a hospital setting is people. Even with the best preventative maintenance and repair service available, it is still people who operate the machinery. Leaders might be surprised to learn how many items of equipment are purchased and used without a formal introduction to the employee. It is the leader's responsibility to be absolutely sure no one uses hospital equipment without being fully orientated to it. Nothing communicates a lack of confidence to a patient better than a staff member who obviously does not know how to use a new item of equipment. Again, hospital leaders should test these systems occasionally on their rounds by asking staff members at random if they know how to use properly the equipment in their areas.

Medical care quality

Who watches out for the medical staff? The obvious answer is that the medical staff watches out for the medical staff. In enlightened hospitals excellent quality accountability systems are set up for this purpose. Some hospitals even have medical staff officers and department chiefs who take their responsibility to monitor the quality of care seriously. However, the hospital CEO and his senior management are also the designated representatives of the board of directors to monitor the quality of care in their institution.

A good reporting system for physician-related problems is essential just as it is for employees. Whether it is an incident report system or some variation, hospital leaders must be aware of physician-related problems as they relate to the quality of care in their institution. Registered nurses are probably the single greatest source of identifying physician-related quality problems. If the hospital CEO and vice president of nursing have carefully made it known to their registered nurses that they want to know about physician problems, problems will surface. Reporting can be further communicated through an active nurse/physician liaison committee that brings to the surface and resolves physician-related quality problems as observed by the nursing staff.

What kind of problems? They are the nitty-gritty problems of day-to-day patient care. The problem of not being able to reach a physician on call. The problem of physician handwriting that is so illegible the registered nurse cannot administer the appropriate medication. The problem of the physician who will not see his patients in ICU promptly after they are admitted. The problem of the physician who will not make rounds every day as good patient care demands.

These are the problems that hospital leaders need to know about, and registered nurses are probably the best source of information.

It behooves the hospital CEO and vice president of nursing to ensure that their RNs know that they will be supported if and when a physician-related problem is identified. Nothing is worse than having a conscientious RN report a problem to the appropriate hospital authority and then have it ignored. This response makes a statement to the staff that quickly discourages any real follow-up for physician problems.

As with employee-related data, patterns sometimes can be evident with physician-related problems. In the case of the poor handwriter, this is likely a problem that has never been dealt with in the physician's career. With physician-related problems, hospital leaders must take action as problems are identified, giving them a thorough review. If, after an appropriate investigation, it is determined that a physician is practicing poor quality care, definite action must be taken. Action of course can range from a friendly warning to dismissal.

Perhaps if hospital leaders had to personally console the families of patients who are receiving poor quality care there would be more attentiveness to physician quality issues. It is a matter of conscience with good hospital leaders. When a problem is identified, hospital leaders should take whatever steps are necessary to protect (and that word is used purposely) the patients from an errant physician. To do otherwise is to sacrifice the trust and perhaps even the well-being of patients entrusted to our care. Some poor quality physicians practice in hospitals. This is a terrible reflection on physicians and hospital leaders. The time is going to come when information about physician quality is much more readily accessible to the public than it is currently. Enlightened leaders will take action long before that day comes. Some may even get fired in the process, but there may be no more noble reason for being fired that the attempted removal of a poor quality physician from the hospital staff.

The impaired physician

It is a fact of life that physicians are practicing in hospitals who are impaired because of alcohol, drug abuse or mental illness. In some cases at least, the hospital's leaders know who the impaired physicians are, but do nothing about them. If a hospital CEO and his senior management know as much about their hospital as they should, they ought to be able to pinpoint all the impaired physicians on their hospital's staff. If they are true leaders, they should do something about those impaired physicians.

What can be done? The first step should be confronting the physician directly and encouraging him to voluntarily seek a leave of absence while gaining appropriate treatment. I know of one upstate New York hospital CEO who has been quite successful with this direct approach. If that does not work, the CEO should initiate formal proceedings to remove the physician from the staff. He should take the leadership position since physicians as a group have demonstrated their unwillingness to do so on countless occasions. The CEO should pursue the issue until the offending physician voluntarily steps down, is unvoluntarily removed from the staff, or no longer is impaired. Allowing impaired physicians to practice in our hospitals is the single greatest disgrace of hospital leaders. Action must be taken to correct this serious problem.

Some concluding thoughts

Hospital leaders are responsible for the quality of care in their hospitals. They can delegate some of the responsibility, but they can never delegate the accountability for that quality. Hospital leaders should know enough about their employees, the equipment, and the physicians in their hospitals to make judgements about their quality. They should have enough courage to do what is right for the patients if there are problems. Even if it means sacrificing their job in the process. After all, if the leaders cannot set the overall quality standards for the hospital, the hospital probably is not worth leading.

PART THREE

LEADERSHIP PARTNERS

CHAPTER FOURTEEN

Wanted: Better Hospital Managers

HOSPITAL LEADERS should recruit and retain the best possible managers. It is the CEO's job to recruit the best senior management, and it is senior management's job to recruit the best department directors and middle management. This occasionally means that people not meeting the criteria of "best" must be separated from the organization. Hospitals have a long way to go to equal their corporate peers in this regard. Keeping people on staff simply because they have contributed in some role for x number of years or are near retirement is a poor leadership approach. It is not acceptable in other industries, nor should it be acceptable in ours. Hospitals must do a better job of weeding out incompetence in their own ranks. If not, the hospital leaders themselves will pay the ultimate price with the loss of their jobs.

The cost based reimbursement system made it possible for hospitals to perform acceptably on a financial basis, even if they were poorly led. There were brilliant exceptions, but mediocrity flourished in an economic environment that yielded a cost plus approach to hospital reimbursement. Those days are gone now, and the challenges faced by current hospitals demand effective management for the hospital to survive and prosper. Recruiting, retaining, and developing hospital management staffs for the future is one of the most exciting aspects of hospital leadership.

Some words about recruiting

Let us begin with some unconventional yet common sensical words of advice on the recruiting process for hospital executives. Hospitals have become an incestuous business. Hospital administration graduate programs produce graduates by the thousands. Some hospitals go so far as to only select management candidates from graduates of the CEO's MHA program. We should not view credentials so narrow mindedly as many hospital leaders currently do.

When hospitals look for a director of housekeeping or dietary, most of them place ads in professional journals and receive hundreds of replies. Five or ten are usually selected for further scrutiny. Then several candidates are interviewed and that is the end of it for most hospitals. They select the individual who best presents himself to the prospective employer. One further step should be added. For executive housekeepers or directors of dietary, what really is important is not how well candidates present themselves in an interview. What is important is how good the food is or how clean the floors are in their current organizations.

For years, I have made it a practice to visit the hospital of a prospective service department head to taste the food and check out the housekeeping. This may seem like overkill; however, it gets to the real nitty-gritty of the candidate's competence. It may be impossible for a prospective executive housekeeper to produce a clean hospital with a new employer if he has not done it in his present hospital. It may be impossible for the director of dietary to produce extremely good food for his new hospital patients if he is not capable of doing it in his current hospital. It is worth the extra time and trouble to visit the candidate's hospital to check on the operation of his or her department. If the candidate passes that test, you can be more certain you are hiring a quality manager.

The same thinking can be applied to most other department head positions and even senior management positions. Finding out what kind of leadership the individual has produced for his or her existing employer is far more enlightening than how polished a candidate is in an interview setting. Personally checking out what the candidate has produced before reaching a final decision is vital. Admittedly, this takes more time and effort and can sometimes get delicate if the candidate's present employer is unaware of his or her intentions. Nevertheless, it is an extremely effective way to tell the difference between a polished interviewee and a true producer.

Another important consideraton when recruiting and evaluating candidates is the spouse, if the candidate has one. Many organizations pay far too little attention to a candidate's spouse. The candidate's spouse should be courted every bit as much as the candidate. The spouse often has an equal say in whether or not the candidate will move. Since many hospitals ignore this, you can separate yourself from the competition by paying extra attention to the spouse. This means hospital tours, interviews, and real estate tours. The more attention hospitals pay to the spouse of an excellent candidate, the better chance they have of landing their first choice, and the better chance you have of retaining the managers if you successfully recruit them.

Evaluating and rewarding

Hospital leaders must know how to set goals and identify expectations for their management staffs. They must have the intellectual toughness to measure performance against those goals and to make the difficult decisions that measurement implies. Part of this is setting appropriate standards for the management staff, and then articulating them to be sure that each member of the staff internalizes them. Having a well-defined performance review system and an articulated set of performance expectations is critical in this regard. A sample of an excellent system is included in Appendix B. A summary of the performance indicators is illustrated in Figure 6.

When performance is less than expected, attempts should be made to improve the performance. After repeated attempts to elevate sub-adequate performance, hospital leaders are faced with the difficult task of separating the erring manager. Although difficult, hospital leaders must understand that if they do not separate the low performers, they themselves are at risk of dismissal, and rightfully so. On the other hand, when performance is exceptional, hospital leaders must recognize and reward performance in a manner that is consistent with the organization's standards and values. This may mean additional responsibilities, more money, more status, or other avenues for recognition of excellence.

Teamwork

Hospital leaders are responsible for forging their staffs into a constructive and effective team. This first means weeding out the incompetent staff members and recruiting and retaining people of the desired level of capability. Then,

FIGURE 6

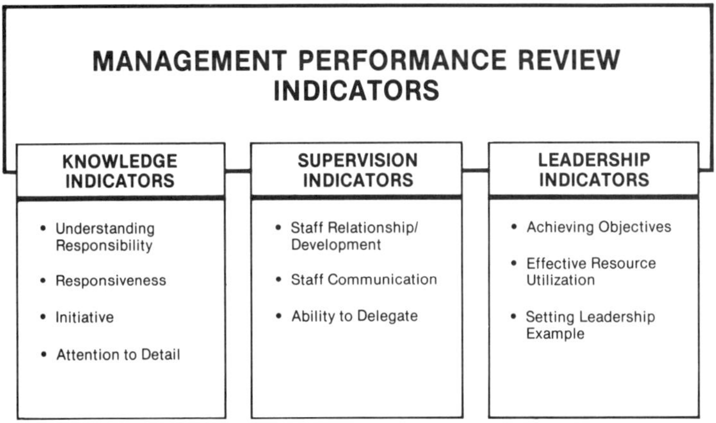
MANAGEMENT PERFORMANCE REVIEW INDICATORS
KNOWLEDGE INDICATORS
• Understanding Responsibility
• Responsiveness
• Initiative
• Attention to Detail
SUPERVISION INDICATORS
• Staff Relationship/ Development
• Staff Communication
• Ability to Delegate
LEADERSHIP INDICATORS
• Achieving Objectives
• Effective Resource Utilization
• Setting Leadership Example

it means incorporating stability. No hospital leader can forge an effective team with a continuous high level of turnover.

One of the most effective examples of forging a cohesive management team is observed in a medium size Wisconsin community hospital. They have evolved a "management council" approach. The CEO and his vice presidents use a collaborative approach to evaluate options and reach key decisions. This is quite different from the more autocratic approach expressed by some CEOs; however, it has performed extremely well.

The successful use of a management council requires a very good teamwork foundation. The key executives rely on each other to fully explore the pros and cons of a given problem or project. For example, this approach has been very effective in prioritizing capital budgets and new staff requests. The CEO is usually confronted with more program requests than resources allow. The management council, as a collaborative group, can rank and prioritize all requests and agree among themselves which should be given higher priority. Sometimes the CEO must referee, but most times the council is able to make the transition from proprietary interests to institutional interests and reach what amounts to research compromises.

Hospital leaders should be teachers

As stated earlier, it is the job of the CEO and senior management to set and communicate corporate values to all employees. It is just as important for hospital leaders to teach and develop their own management staffs. It is time-consuming and requires commitment. But if Jan Carlson could personally train 2000 SAS managers during that company's turnaround, hospital leaders can certainly devote the time and energy to training their considerably smaller management staffs.

The CEO should be the primary teacher for management, supplemented by senior management and outside "experts". The use of outside experts should be minimized. Many hospital leaders delegate management training to consultants. They are missing a tremendous opportunity to instill their vision and passion directly to managers. One Wisconsin hospital CEO uses an annual spring lecture series consisting of six to eight three-hour presentations of importance to the organization. Subjects included such practical topics as employee evaluations, capital budget preparation, attention to detail, marketing, etc. The CEO usually teaches half of the programs and uses his senior managers for the rest. Only rarely are outside trainers used, and then only for topics of such technical nature that no one inside the organization could present them effectively.

Another related approach used by the same Wisconsin hospital is to purchase a timely management book for each member of the middle and senior management. The book is then used as the subject of an annual management retreat. For example, a copy of *A Passion for Excellence* was purchased for each department director and vice president and then used for a retreat to create hospital applications for the successful management approaches discussed in the book. These types of working retreats, based on a particularly good book, can stimulate creativity and develop new approaches to leading hospitals more effectively.

In the final analysis, the quality of a hospital's management team is going to reflect the interest and commitment of its leaders. If the CEO and senior management do not think training and development are important enough to do personally, then they should expect to preside over a mediocre group. If, on the other hand, they see teaching their management staff as a priority worthy of their personal efforts, they will be rewarded with a management group that reflects the leader's values, expertise and commitment.

CHAPTER FIFTEEN

Leading the Board

CAN YOU IMAGINE the chief executive officer of a 20 million dollar corporation asking the board to select carpet for the lobby in the company's headquarters? Can you imagine a corporate chief executive encouraging the board to participate in the selection decisions for middle management? Can you imagine a corporation board which sees as its responsibility meeting with disgruntled production workers? If you are a corporate board member you would not even think of participating in these decisions. However, if you are a hospital board member, you may think it is your duty to participate in such decisions.

An effective hospital leader would not think of letting his board select carpet for the hospital lobby. But hospital boards participate in decisions like this every month in hospitals around the country. Why? There are many reasons, but primary among them is the lack of leadership in hospitals and boards. It is the hospital CEO's job to change this climate and create a new one in which the board functions as a policy-making body and the CEO and senior management operate the corporation on a day-to-day basis. Richard Umbdenstock says "the CEO should be the initiator, the motivator, and the implementor, but at the same time the CEO must provide the board with the proper tools for the same kind of sound decision making the board expects of the management team.''[11]

Creating the role of the hospital board

The two most important jobs for a hospital board are, one, selecting the chief executive officer, and two, evaluating and retaining the CEO if he or she is an effective leader. The next most important job is firing an ineffective hospital leader. It is not the hospital board's role to directly manage the operations of a hospital. And yet so many boards are involved in so many operating decisions that it is no wonder hospital CEOs come and go so quickly.

The hospital CEO should lead the board. When an effective hospital leader has been hired and retained, that leader needs to establish the role of the chief executive officer. This role should be no different from the chief executive officer of any comparably sized corporation. That means that the board sets policy, allocates resources, and leaves the operation of the corporation to its CEO and senior management. This does not happen by accident. A few boards around the country have enlightened leadership and they set an excellent example for the rest of us.

Unfortunately, this is not the norm. The hospital CEO must be the driving force to change the governance climate if the board sees its role as managing operations rather than setting policy. If done effectively, the hospital leader will establish with his board several important roles in addition to selecting, evaluating, and retaining the chief executive. Basically, the role of the board, beyond hiring and retaining the CEO, is threefold: overseeing the quality of medical care; strategic planning for the hospital's future; and major resource allocation decisions.

Notice that selecting carpet and interviewing employees were not mentioned. Nor was setting salaries for middle management or hiring administrative staff members. These are the roles of the hospital CEO and they must clearly and strongly establish this in their organization.

Evaluating the performance of the CEO is a key responsibility of the board. The first step in setting up an effective evaluation process is clearly defining expectations and responsibilities. Beyond that, a well-defined evaluation process is a must. Many boards are moving away from an informal process, which involves no more than an annual salary review, to a formal process. The CEO can be the catalyst for developing a good evaluation process, since it is clearly in the CEO's and the hospital's best interest to do so. Use of a CEO evaluation committee is gaining acceptance in some hospitals. A sample CEO evaluation policy is attached in Appendix D, which describes in detail the process used by a Wisconsin community hospital and now being adopted for use by other midwest hospital boards. The evaluation process is illustrated graphically in Figure 8 (p. 158).

A footnote about board committees. Too many committees exist. With an effective hospital CEO and senior management most of these traditional committees are simply not needed. Why should a hospital have a building and grounds committee if it has an effective chief executive who knows when to replace the roof and when its time for a boiler overhaul? Why should a hospital board have a personnel committee? The chief executive should be able to administer personnel policy and employee discipline as necessary. These are just a few of the outdated committees that populate many boards today and do nothing to further the interest of the hospital. They continue to exist because of weak leadership in hospitals, not because of a serious need for their existence.

What does leading the board mean?

Leading the board means establishing the role of the CEO of the corporation. That means establishing a clearly defined set of responsibilities in the form of a job description or clearly defined description of duties in the corporation bylaws. At a minimum, these defined responsibilities should include: board development; planning; recruitment of the management and professional staff; human resource management; overseeing the quality of medical care; allocation of resources; regulatory compliance; and promotion of the corporation. A sample detailed job description for the chief executive officer is included in Appendix C. A graphic representation of CEO roles is illustrated in Figure 7. Selecting board members is another aspect of leading the board. In non-hospital corporations, the CEO is the key element in board member selection. Of course, there may be a nominating committee, but it is the CEO who does most of the evaluation of potential board members and makes selection recommendations. In hospitals, it should be no different. The CEO should be the primary individual to identify potential board member candidates, to evaluate their prospective contribution, and to recommend new board members as positions open.

Evaluating existing board members and committees is also a function of the hospital leadership. This must be done together with the board leadership, but the hospital CEO should take the initiative to ensure that there is an adequate

FIGURE 7

CHIEF EXECUTIVE OFFICER RESPONSIBILITIES

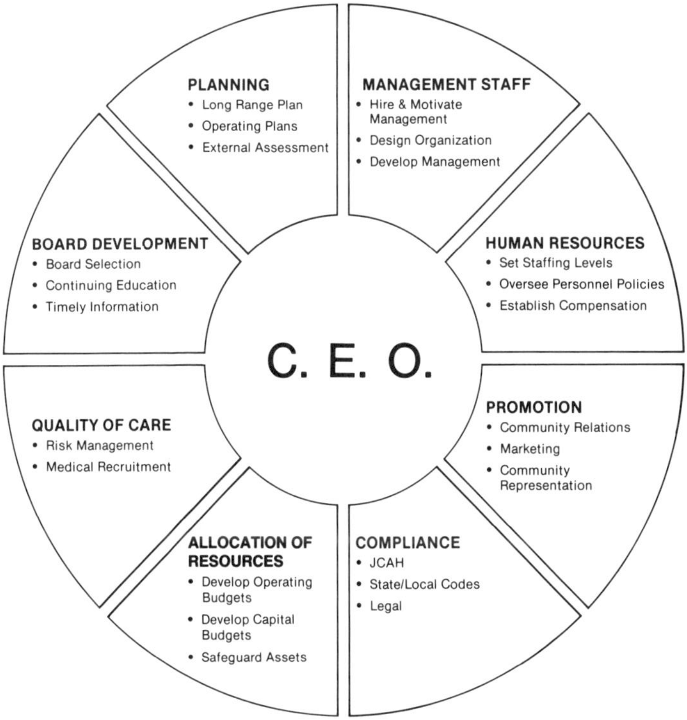

FIGURE 8

CEO EVALUATION

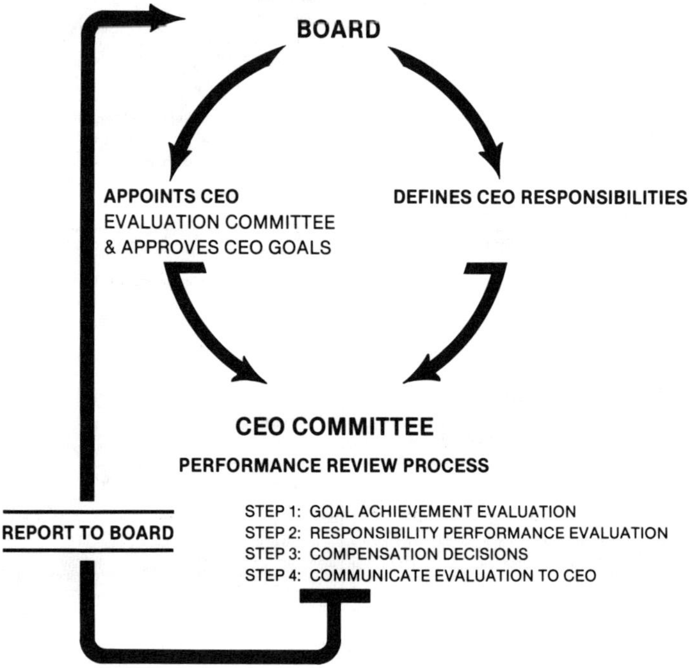

process for evaluating individual board members and the effectiveness of all board committees. This can be touchy at times; however, the CEO must accomplish it. To do less would be to ignore one important aspect of his responsibilities.

Developing individual members of the board and making the board a cohesive decision making unit is also a responsibility of the hospital CEO. Arranging for educational programs, whether they be medical presentations, managerial presentations, consultant presentations or trips to various seminars available for board members is very important. It is also important, along with the selection process, to develop the overall capabilities of the hospital board. This means evaluating the various strengths and weaknesses represented on the hospital board and recruiting, as necessary, new board members to fill the weak spots.

A tremendous time void is created as hospital boards, with the aid of effective leaders, are moving away from hands-on operating bodies to policy-making corporate boards. The extra time that used to be spent deciding on the lobby carpet must be better used elsewhere. Effective hospital leaders are finding ways to use their board members as consultants. This can be on special projects in areas of board member expertise. Of course, it sometimes blurs the line between policy and operations when board members are used as consultants, but the effective leader will be able to shoulder this risk and gain maximum potential from his board members as consultants and advisors.

Leading board meetings

Another important role for the hospital CEO is to lead board meetings. This includes developing agendas, planning meetings, and serving as principle speaker and presenter at board meetings. Many boards have very rigid rules for conducting business. This means that the agenda arrangement is always the same, no matter what the issues. Sometimes this means leaving the most important items for discussion to the very end, under "new business," when attention is at its lowest. Hospital CEOs need to develop priority based agendas where the most critical items are discussed first, leaving routine business for last. Progressive boards change their meeting agenda sequence frequently, putting the most important agenda items first and leaving routine reporting duties and committee reports until last.

Any CEO who allows time to be wasted reading committee minutes in a board meeting should be drawn and quartered. All committee minutes and reports should be distributed at least several days before the meeting to allow ample time for review.

Some hospital leaders make the mistake of routinely bringing a passle of subordinates to board meetings to make presentations. Although this is a matter of personal choice, I believe the most effective hospital CEOs interact with their board members solo. It is an important aspect of hospital leadership that the board sees its contact as the CEO, not other management subordinates. This does not mean that senior management should never attend a board meeting or talk to board members, but it does mean that the hospital CEO should be knowledgeable enough to present the monthly financial statements, the various operating and capital budgets and similar matters of critical importance to the corporation. There is no reason to rely on a chief financial officer or other senior manager to do that work.

Finally, the CEO and board leadership should work to make the board meetings interesting. By interesting I do not mean carrying a free for all discussion about what color to paint the x-ray department. Instead, I mean varying the routine occasionally to include hospital tours, "field trips" to other health-related organizations, and timely educational presentations. Board leadership and the CEO should create a flexible program that satisfies the need for the board to be thoroughly informed, and at the same time achieves a high level of interest and professional standardization to board members. A well thought out program of board development can help achieve this important balance.

Board development

The subject of board development conjures up different images to different people. On one extreme, a hospital can expend so much energy on "educating" its board that directors with time constraints "tune out." On the other extreme, some hospitals spend no effort at all to enhance their board members' understanding of medicine and the health care environment.

One good development approach is to set aside thirty minutes or so in each meeting to conduct a continuing education session. Board members and the CEO should select the topics to be presented. The CEO can then make the arrangements for appropriate speakers and the meetings can begin with the education session. This approach was modeled after the monthly medical staff meeting approach used by a Wisconsin community hospital. It presents timely and informative subjects within a time frame which does not intrude too much on a board member's time.

One way to integrate board development and planning board meetings, as suggested by governance consultant Richard Umbdenstock, is to develop an annual board calendar. The calendar has several components: recurring board agenda items, special topics, and board development presentations.

Recurring item examples are budget reviews, medical staff appointments, meetings. Special items are discussions or presentations contributing to effective review and decision making by the board. For example, if the board is going to decide on replacing a CT scanner in November as part of the capital budget review, perhaps an update on CT technology delivered by the hospital's radiologists in September would be in order.

Board development topics can be presented by inside "experts" like physicians and senior managers, or by outside consultants. Examples might be a presentation on HMOs, medical malpractice, advances in cardiology technology, or legal issues in governance. The board should be polled prior to the beginning of the year to determine its preference for development topics. Their interests, along with the input from the CEO, will determine the topics for presentation during the year. The calendar should be completed and distributed to all board members at the beginning of each year. A well executed board calendar is an invaluable tool to the CEO and board chairman for planning meeting agendas during the year.

A sample annual board calendar for a community hospital board is shown in Figure 9.

As a supplement to this approach, an annual retreat to review in depth a subject of great importance can also be effective in developing the board. Retreats are best done "off-site," away from the hospital, and can be combined with a social event to include board members' spouses. Most hospitals do not pay board members for their valuable time,

FIGURE 9

SAMPLE ANNUAL BOARD MEETING CALENDAR

BOARD MEETING	RECURRING ITEMS	DEVELOPMENT TOPICS
JANUARY	MEDICAL STAFF REAPPOINTMENT	LEGAL ISSUES IN GOVERNANCE
FEBRUARY		HMO/PPO PRESENTATION
MARCH	ANNUAL FINANCIAL AUDIT	OVERVIEW OF FUTURE TECHNOLOGY
APRIL	ANNUAL CORPORATION MEETING	TRENDS IN GOVERNANCE
MAY		BOARD MEMBER EVALUATION
JUNE		CAPITAL MARKET ACCESS
JULY		TRENDS IN HOSPITAL REIMBURSEMENT
AUGUST		MEDICAL STAFF CREDENTIALING
SEPTEMBER		MARKET RESEARCH OVERVIEW
OCTOBER	OPERATING BUDGET REVIEW	TRENDS IN RISK MANAGEMENT
NOVEMBER	CAPITAL BUDGET REVIEW	NEW VENTURE DEVELOPMENT
DECEMBER	BOARD MEMBER REAPPOINTMENT	MALPRACTICE OVERVIEW

so a day or two away annually can become a nice perk for board members in addition to providing an educational opportunity.

Lastly, excellent board education seminars are available around the country on timely subjects, and the CEO should look for programs that can enhance the understanding of individual board members on subjects of interest to the hospital.

A few words about boardmanship

Every hospital leader is going to be faced at one time or another with a meddling board member. This is someone who complains about their neighbor's care in the middle of a board meeting or perhaps someone who intercedes on behalf of an employee who was fired. An effective hospital leader deals with this type of problem firmly and establishes that the board room and board meetings are places to discuss matters of policy, not individual problems and complaints. These subjects should be addressed directly to the hospital CEO in private.

It takes a particularly strong leader to establish and enforce this policy; however, it is important to do so. I would not recommend going as far as one New York CEO did several years ago when confronted with a personnel matter during a board meeting. That CEO calmly reached into his pocket and extracted the keys to his office and announced that if any member of the board felt better qualified to resolve issues of that type they were welcome to occupy his office. No one reached for the keys. Without being as extreme, an effective CEO does have the courage to constructively tell a board member to keep the board meetings for policy discussions, not for problem review. Doing so will elevate the board meetings beyond a discussion of small details and personal agendas to the realm of policy setting.

Mutual trust and respect

The CEO and board should work hard to achieve mutual trust and respect. As stated earlier, the CEO should lead the board. At the same time the CEO should keep the board well informed, using it in a fashion that maximizes its contributions to the hospital. This is not easy. Lines are sometimes drawn and the management versus policy "turf" is sometimes argued.

Effective hospital and board leaders will be able to get beyond the turf struggles and forge effective partnerships. The days of boards selecting lobby carpets are drawing to an end. I am confident that boards will find their new roles as policy makers more interesting and more fulfilling.

CHAPTER SIXTEEN

Physicians: It's Time to Lead Them, Too

MORE HOSPITAL LEADERS have probably been dismissed because of problems with physicians than for any other single reason. As a consultant once mused, most boards just find it easier to replace a chief executive than an established cardiologist with a busy hospital practice. In many hospitals, there exists an ongoing war between the hospital leaders and members of the medical staff. It is definitely true that hospital interests and physician interests frequently are in conflict. It is also true that hospital leaders need to look more carefully for a common ground so they are less susceptible to threats of being fired due to problems with their physicians.

The growing use of contracts and termination agreements for hospital leaders has helped to reduce hospital leader firings because of physician whim. Hospital leaders can be more courageous and forthright when they have a contract allowing for payment of a year's salary if they are fired. Regardless of the source of courage, hospital leaders are increasingly facing off with physicians successfully. More importantly, enlightened leaders are looking for ways to enhance the physician-leader partnership in ways that will further their mutual interests. There is a definite change and improvement in terms of hospital and physician relationships. That improvement will make it easier for both groups to succeed in a competitive environment.

Education is the key

Hospital leaders need to take the initiative in helping physicians understand the competitive environment. They do not teach marketing in medical school. In fact, some cynics might suggest that the training of physicians precludes developing good patient relations skills.

A hospital cannot be successful in a competitive environment unless physicians are part of the service focus on customer and patient relations. Regardless of how effective hospital leaders are in teaching their staffs good customer relation skills, they will ultimately fail to achieve their full organization potential unless physicians are part of the team.

Education and setting a good example are the keys to achieving good results with physicians. Hospital leaders should introduce their physicians to marketing through presentations on subjects such as marketing physician practices and increasing patient satisfaction. There are excellent physician and management consultants who can present very effective programs for medical staffs. These programs stress practical advice like listening to patients, not rushing through office visits, and making follow-up phone calls on a timely basis. They also cover such topics as office waiting time management, patient scheduling systems, and accessibility for emergency conditions.

Hospital leaders also should remember that the changes in reimbursement systems are very disruptive to physicians.

Thus, provide good education programs for the medical staff so that procedures such as discharge planning and preadmission screenings are understood.

Additionally, hospital leaders should set a good example for their physicians. It does no good for a CEO to preach customer satisfaction skills to his physicians when he presides over a surly group of nurses and an uncooperative management team. Beyond education, hospital leaders can use many other progressive approaches to work more effectively with their physicians.

Identify the stars

Just as some hospital leaders are more intelligent and more effective than others, so it is with physicians. One opportunity for hospital leaders is to identify the "stars." The stars are physicians of superior quality who contribute in a major way to the success of the facility. It is not that difficult to identify physician stars. Training, commitment to continuing education, hard work, and high rates of success in diagnosis and treatment are easily determined by hospital leaders. Although it does take a certain amount of subjective judgement, this analysis should not be difficult for well-informed leaders.

Once physician stars are identified, hospital leaders need to assist those physicians to succeed in any way they can. This may mean allocating resources, developing new facilities and services that enhance the star's training and capabilities, and promoting the star's potential contributions to the hospital and medical community. Does this sound more like Hollywood than hospitals? Perhaps. However, even large hospitals' fortunes can rise or fall on the backs of a small number of physicians. Enlightened hospital leaders do everything they can to maximize the contribution of these special physicians to their hospital.

Parking lots and donut fights

I know one hospital CEO who constantly picks gratuitous fights with physicians. He spends part of his day denying requests from physicians to have donuts in their morning meetings or to eat lunch in the hospital auditorium during educational conferences. The CEO instills that attitude in his senior management as well, so there are usually several ongoing skirmishes, like how long the medical staff library door should be open or whether or not the chairs in the physician dictation booths need to be replaced. It is true the hospital is saving money. It is also true the hospital is winning battles at the cost of losing the war in terms of establishing constructive relationships with its physicians.

Physicians should be treated as if they were guests in a high class hotel. Not only should they get donuts and coffee at physician meetings if they desire, they should get bagels and cream cheese if they ask for it. Although luncheon meetings may not meet the Ritz-Carlton standards, they should be as good as any local restaurant. Education programs should provide gourmet delights in the hope that they will attract a few more physicians. The quality of the food is an important factor in getting physicians to attend meetings. The better the food, the higher the attendance.

Parking may be the single biggest source of irritation experienced by physicians. Give physicians the best parking spaces available and be sure there are enough. If that means some employees have to walk a few extra steps, so be it. Employees do not medically treat patients. Give your physicians a nice lounge, serve them good food, and above all give them choice parking spaces. While this may not guarantee a satisfactory physician-leader relationship, it does not hurt!

Marketing your physicians

Most physicians today still look upon advertising as something that is reserved for used cars and pantyhose. But the fact is, advertising and marketing are here to stay in the hospital industry. It is also true that the reputation of one's physicians is probably the single greatest factor in determining the hospital's reputation. Therefore, hospital leaders must determine ways to effectively promote their highly skilled physicians.

A good physician, of course, is in the eye of the beholder. Good may refer to bedside manner, clinical competence, appearance, or a combination thereof. The good qualities of the chosen physicians should be used to promote the medical community and the hospital.

How can this be done? The best way is gaining face to face community exposure for your good physicians. Convincing a busy vascular surgeon to give a talk to the Women's Garden Club or a busy orthopedic surgeon to give a talk about athletic injuries to local coaches is not easy. But it can be done. It helps to do all of the staff work. That means preparing the slides, researching the subject matter, taking care of the slide projectors, and even driving the physician to and from the talk.

As mentioned earlier, effective hospital leaders need to instruct their physicians in the value of marketing. Enlightened hospital leaders know that marketing is more than advertising. Hospitals need to teach physicians more about market research, community preferences, selection criteria for hospitals and physicians, and the effectiveness of various approaches in improving the reputation of physicians and hospitals.

Involving physicians in marketing planning and promotion can also contribute greatly to the hospital's success. This does not mean that hospital leaders should let physicians write advertising copy. This would be the worst use of physician time imaginable. Most physicians will write advertising copy that only another physician or nuclear physicist can understand. Let the advertising pros do their work.

Other successful approaches to marketing physicians include encouraging physicians to develop office "newsletters" or to write a health care column for the local newspaper. The hospital can help by writing news releases highlighting physician accomplishments and arranging T.V. and radio coverage when new physicians are recruited or new services introduced. By working with physicians, hospital leaders can achieve substantial promotion of these physicians without having them feel as if they are lowering their professional dignity by advertising.

Physician recruiting

This is a difficult subject for some hospital leaders. Some leaders think it is the job of physicians to recruit other physicians. Not so. Hospital leaders must realize that recruiting is a joint task of the hospital and its physicians. Sometimes, it will even be necessary for hospital leaders to recruit new physicians over the objections of existing ones. This may be necessary because of quality problems, it may be necesary because of attitudinal problems, and/or it may be necessary because the addition of new specialists is more in the interest of the hospital than the existing medical staff.

It is virtually impossible for a hospital leader to recruit without some physician assistance, but hospitals can take the initiative and leadership role in recruiting. There are all sorts of way to recruit, ranging from search firms to residency contacts to advertisements. Hospital leaders have to select the approach that is best suited for the open position and the resources available to recruiting.

When interviewing, remember hospitals are interviewing the spouse as well as the physician. The effective recruiter makes sure that the spouse is treated as well if not better than the physician candidate. Traveling to the candidate's home base can be a very effective tool in competitive physician recruiting. One hospital CEO charters planes to fly groups of physicians and their spouses to visit prospective physicians in their home community. Chartered planes make a dramatic statement of interest and can be a very effective use of both the hospital leader and the physicians' time.

Hospital leaders should identify the prospective physician's needs and then have the courage to recruit the physician even if the existing medical staff is lukewarm or in opposition. They must do what is right for their hospital and their patient population, even if this means accepting conflict with existing physicians.

Responsiveness

Hospital leaders should always be responsive to problems of and opportunities for their physicians. They should have the ability to give answers, make decisions, and communicate quickly. Many hospital leaders sink into trouble because they are unable or afraid to make negative decisions when it concerns physicians. Physicians are like board members and employees. They want answers and they want them quickly, not in six months. Hospital leaders should be sensitive to this and should also have the courage to give negative as well as positive responses.

A Long Island hospital has a system of administrative rounds with physicians that uniquely enhances communication and responsiveness between management and physicians. Each senior member of the management staff makes rounds once a week with a key admitting physician. The dialogue generated does a great deal to resolve small irritating problems for the physician and gives the hospital leaders the opportunity to respond directly to the needs of their key physicians.

Although all hospital leaders have subordinates, dealing with physicians is something that should not be delegated too low in the organization, particularly with reference to chronic complainers and superstars. When a star physician wants something, leaders should do their best to deliver. Fast. Of course this may not always be possible, but it is always possible to get an answer back to the requesting physician or someone experiencing a problem. Of course, it works both ways. Whenever a problem surfaces with a physician through the community or his patients, hospital leaders have an obligation to communicate that directly to the physician as quickly as possible. Hospital leaders also have an obligation to get back quickly with an answer.

Physicians should know the hospital leader's expectations with reference to communication. It should be known that cocktail party "back stabbing" is unacceptable and that it diminishes the credibility of the offending physician. In other words, the hospital leader should establish with his physicians that the best form of communication is face to face, not through third parties and not through politically expedient mechanisms. Most hospital leaders have medical staffs that are small enough to allow a direct form of communication which is manageable and more satisfying to both parties.

Teach them well

I once heard a physician remark that physicians are no longer educable after they reach the age of 35. Such folly is worth disproving. The monthly medical staff meeting or executive committee is an opportunity to familiarize physicians with upcoming events and the financial status of the hospital. It also provides a source of input and feedback for the leader. Of course, this carries some risk. Some medical staff meetings resemble the Vietnam War more than a gathering of well-educated professionals. Not withstanding the barbs and the gratuitous criticisms that occasionally fly in both directions, hospital leaders can and should continuously try to educate their physicians about what is going on in the external environment and in the hospital.

The end result of that understanding can be a physician-hospital partnershp focusing on better patient care outcomes rather than posturing and guerrilla warfare.

CHAPTER SEVENTEEN

On Leading Volunteers

VOLUNTEER organizations can be an extremely positive or extremely negative force in a hospital environment. Volunteers must be led to the extent that they internalize the same corporate values as hospital employees. This is no easy task. It requires courage and determination. It should be noted that "crossing" volunteer or auxiliary organizations has certainly gotten more than one hospital CEO fired. On the other hand, not providing direction and leadership to volunteer organizations can harm a hospital's reputation and diminish its ability to provide excellent services. Leadership for volunteers is a tricky proposition, but if done properly it can produce an environment where volunteers have the opportunity to be personally fulfilled while performing valuable services to hospital patients.

The quality of individual volunteers and volunteer organizations varies with the hospital and community. Each volunteer organization has its own individual character and therein lies the dilemma. A volunteer organization can be extremely beneficial for the hospital and community. On the other hand, it can become an extremely detrimental force if not appropriately channeled. In the worst cases, volunteer organizations live up to Mark Twain's prediction that "sometimes what you get for free is worth the price." If that happens, hospital leaders have no one to blame but themselves.

The necessity to lead volunteer organizations is a foreign concept in many hospitals. They lead themselves. They operate under a different set of rules from other parts of the hospital, and they frequently have a political component that many hospital leaders either fail to understand or are so afraid to "offend" that they take a hands off approach.

Volunteers should be led, and it is the job of the CEO and senior management to do the leading. This requires some courage and a willingness to make unpopular decisions on occasion. Sometimes those decisions might make volunteers mad. Some might even quit or, heaven forbid, write a nasty letter to the board or local newspaper. On the other hand, firm leadership can create an environment where volunteers are completely in tune with the rest of the organization and helping fulfill its mission, rather than simply providing a place for well-intentioned volunteers to spend some time.

An example of the "tough decisions" that need to be faced with leading volunteers is deciding where volunteers can be most helpful to the hospital and where their presence may be detrimental.

The front desk example

Many hospitals have lobby reception desks staffed by volunteers. This is an example of a volunteer assignment fraught with potential difficulty. The front desk is the first impression a patient or visitor receives upon arriving in a hospital. The quality of that first exchange sets the tone for all others that follow.

By nature, volunteers are part-time workers. Becoming totally familiar with all hospital services and operations is just not practical for each volunteer. Even some small hospitals have twenty or more volunteers serving at one time or another on front desk duty. Additionally, with such a large group of volunteers staffing the front desk, it is difficult for each of them to display a consistently good attitude toward visitors and patients.

Volunteers consider the front desk assignment one of the best available, a "plum." They get to see what is going on and are highly visible to the community. However, as some hospitals have learned, front desk volunteers sometimes violate confidentiality and present a less than positive image to the public. This can create a poor first impression.

The hospital front desk is not the best place for volunteers. The reception function is one of the most important in the hospital and should not be left to volunteers whose expertise and attitudes cannot be consistently dependable. Hospital leaders who have volunteers on their front desk should "bite the bullet" and replace them with receptionists. In the short run, you may anger some volunteers by this move. In the long run, hospitals will be better serving their customers.

Selecting volunteers

Selection, evaluation and even disciplining volunteers may be new concepts for some hospital leaders. Many hospitals' selection criteria for volunteers is to accept all comers. The sad fact is that many volunteer organizations have members who are incapable of performing their assigned job. The selection of volunteers is as important as selecting employees for the organization. This means completing appropriate applications, conducting interviews to determine interests and attitudes, and critically evaluating what the individual can contribute to the hospital. If minimum criteria are not met, prospective volunteers should be turned away.

Orientating and evaluating volunteers

After selection, volunteers should be oriented thoroughly to the hospital. It is recommended that new volunteers attend orientation classes for new employees. That will give them an effective orientation to the hospital in general. In addition, they should be specifically oriented to their assigned responsibilities. This can be jointly done by the volunteer director and the department director in the area in which the volunteer will serve. The orientation process should stress behavior as well as performance expectations.

Evaluation of volunteers is also very important, but it may be a new concept to some hospitals. The lack of evaluation standards is clearly evident in many hospitals. How can you tell? Just look around for the 78-year-old volunteer who is hard of hearing and sitting at the front desk having difficulty hearing patients and visitors and forgetting where three quarters of the departments are in the hospital. There should be minimum performance standards for all volunteers, similar in nature to those set for employees. When volunteers no longer meet minimum standards, they should be retired or reassigned to areas where they can meet appropriate minimum standards. This may seem harsh, but it is simply good judgement. Our patients and community judge all people that they meet in our hospitals. If we allow volunteers to perform functions for which they are unqualified, they should be removed from those positions.

Lastly, we need to touch on the issue of disciplining volunteers. Many hospital leaders take the position that they cannot discipline someone who contributes their time for free. Nothing is further from the truth. Volunteers should be held accountable to the same basic standards as employees. When those standards are not met, some form of discipline should be applied. This should include "terminating" the volunteer for sustained poor performance or poor attitude. To do otherwise can significantly compromise the hospital's image and its performance.

Can volunteers accept change?

Volunteer organizations tend to be made up of senior citizens. This group may be less likely and less inclined to change than employee groups or even medical staffs. Herein lies the challenge for hospital leaders. They must persuade volunteer organizations to change as the hospital business changes. We are in one of the most rapidly changing environments our industry has ever experienced. Employees and physicians are making the transition; volunteer organizations must do likewise. It is the responsibility of hospital leaders to inform volunteer organizations, both in groups and perhaps even individually, of the need for change.

Many volunteer organizations have accepted change constructively by integrating volunteer efforts with hospital marketing programs, inventing new fund raising approaches, and creating new services to complement the changing nature of hospital care. An innovative Illinois hospital uses volunteers to sponsor an annual summer "Baby Homecoming" picnic for children born at the hospital in the last five years and their parents. This well-attended event is integrated with the hospital's marketing efforts for its excellent maternity services.

A Georgia hospital created a "Love Light" program to raise funds for the hospital each Christmas season. The volunteers sell Christmas tree lights in memory of loved ones and have a special lighting ceremony. This has become a social highlight during the Christmas season. Not only has this program become one of the volunteers' most successful annual fund raising events, it has also created an opportunity for all members of the community, no matter how financially disadvantaged, to participate in hospital giving.

Many hospital volunteer organizations have funded and staffed "Lifeline" programs for their community hospitals. These programs, which permit homebound community members to be tied directly to the hospital emergency room via a communication link, have been very successful in helping re-orient hospitals from an exclusively acute care focus to a more community-oriented health care facility.

On the other hand, some hospitals allow themselves to be held captive by rigid volunteer organizations and outdated programs. Staffing reception desks, selling local art work, and running the switchboard are good examples. Their leaders must be strong enough to accept the fact that some "old line" volunteers may never change and remove them from their organizations. Just because volunteers work for free does not give them license to second guess and critique the hospital's direction.

Volunteer recognition

There are many built-in opportunities for hospital leaders to recognize and praise their volunteers. Virtually all hospitals have annual recognition dinners and other monthly or annual events providing great opportunities to praise individual volunteers and the efforts of the group as a whole. Hospital leaders should not delegate this communication to subordinates. Volunteer leaders need to receive that recognition directly from the top of the organization. Hospital leaders can also use these occasions to keep their volunteers informed about significant changes in the hospital industry and to challenge them with new ways of responding to the changes.

Keeping volunteer leaders informed is also extremely important. This can be effectively accomplished through an informal luncheon every several months that informs the volunteer leaders of major upcoming plans for the hospital, and how the volunteer organization fits in with those plans. It also can be a great opportunity for hospital leaders to reinforce the corporate values and the expectations for volunteers with reference to those values.

Some concluding thoughts

It is widely recognized that volunteers can be an extremely positive force for a hospital. Less known is that volunteers can be a negative force. Hospital leaders, to gain the most advantage from their volunteers, should take a more aggressive position leading their volunteers. They must be willing to accept some tensions and establish selection and evaluation criteria similar to that for employees.

As a parting word of advice, the hospital leader must lead his volunteers, not be led by them. The old expression of "having the tail wag the dog" comes to mind when thinking of volunteer organizations. In well-led hospitals, the dog is still wagging the tail.

CHAPTER EIGHTEEN

The Future of Hospital Leadership

THE VIEW of hospital leadership presented here is somewhat more basic than what is currently being espoused. A back to the basics approach is what is needed in today's hospital. Some will conclude that this approach is going backward rather than forward. What is fundamentally important in hospitals are the patients, and whether or not they get better. The sophistication of our computers and the complexity of our organization structures is not what is important. Here are a few predictions about hospital leadership.

Community not-for-profit hospitals

To hear some futurists talk, you would think that by 1990 there will be no more independent not-for-profit community hospitals. To paraphrase Mark Twain, predictions of their demise are greatly exaggerated. Although the growth of for-profit chains and not-for-profit chains is impressive, it will slow in the last half of this decade. The fundamental reason for this is there will be better quality leadership in not-for-profit community hospitals. With better quality leadership, community hospitals will prosper and probably even surpass their for-profit counterparts in terms of organizational, financial and quality of care performance.

Behind this prediction is an optimism for the quality of hospital leadership. In a not-for-profit community hospital, the position of chief executive is the highest position of leadership. With more enlightened boards and better quality leaders, community hospitals will become like their business sector counterparts. Aggressive and highly competent leaders will be attracted to community hospital positions in a very competitive and financially demanding marketplace. Boards will pay these leaders more and reward them consistent with similarly sized business organizations.

On the other hand, the job of hospital CEO is the lowest job on the totem pole of the large for-profit and not-for-profit chains. It is a starting point for the move upward through corporate structure. With this in mind, the job of hospital CEO in either the for-profit or not-for-profit chains is not seen as an end in itself; instead it is seen as a starting point for a corporate career. This leads to high turnover and younger and more inexperienced leaders at the hospital CEO level. These people will be be outperformed every time by strong and capable leaders in the community hospital setting who see the CEO job as an end in itself.

Diversification

A vertical and horizontal diversification craze is currently going on in hospitals. You cannot attend regional or national hospital gatherings without at least some meetings on the subject of diversification. It is certainly in vogue now for hospital leaders to get involved with businesses, some related and some not related to their basic hospital mission. This craze will decline substantially by the end of this decade. Why? For the same reason that diversification is declining in industry.

In the last two decades there has been a craze for diversification through acquisitions. Many large conglomerates have later found themselves unable to run profitably the many businesses they acquired. Divestiture has been the standard mode of some of these diversified conglomerates during this decade. Companies are getting back to the basics and sticking with the businesses they know how to run well. Hospital leaders are going to come to the same realization that their corporate counterparts came to. That is, if you cannot run it, do not buy it or start it.

Networks and systems

Networks and systems are much in vogue today. Voluntary Hospitals of America, American Health Systems, and many others have enjoyed phenomenal growth in the past decade. That growth is going to slow as hospital leaders begin to examine the real economic payoffs for belonging to a system.

What are the benefits? Some say group purchasing; but hospitals can enjoy the results of group purchasing less expensively than belonging to a national network. Some say access to pre-screened consultants. But intelligent leaders are smart enough to screen and select their own consultants. Some say there is great strength in numbers. Nonsense. The greatest strength a hospital can have is to produce good outcomes for its customers, and no national group is going to accomplish that for its individual members. Some say that access to capital is the reason to be part of a system. I say that any well-run community hospital will have access to all of the capital it can use.

As the quality of leadership is increased in hospitals, the need to be part of a network will decline. Effective leaders will do well in their own marketplace without the expense of belonging to a network. In fact, hospital leaders of the future will resist the notion of networks because of the prohibitive costs and the lack of real benefits for their individual hospitals.

Hospital financial performance

A lot of doom and gloom is forecast for hospitals. Prospective payment, utilization review, and other forms of financial restrictions are afflicting hospitals in an ever-increasing force. For the most part, these forces will ultimately benefit the hospitals as well as the general public. They are forcing us to manage more effectively.

For years, hospitals had it just like defense contractors. Cost plus was the name of the game. Now those days are over and we are beginning to learn how to run our hospitals as our counterparts in industry run their corporations. This means hospitals are buying more effectively, building more effectively, and paying more attention to customers' wants and needs. The financial performance of hospitals is eventually going to improve tremendously for those hospitals that survive. There will be a number of hospitals that will be victims of the current competitive squeeze. But for the first time our industry is being subjected to the rigors of the survival of the fittest. That will produce some successful examples of excellent financial management in hospitals. We can manage our hospitals a lot better than we have in the past, and with good leadership we are going to do just that.

On computers

Hospitals have gone overboard on computers. The first to realize it were the for-profit chains. Whenever they purchase or sign a new management contract for a new hospital, one of the first moves is usually to streamline and downsize the computer operation.

No one would disagree that there will always be a place for computers in hospitals. However, the days of the large mainframes are numbered because hospital leaders are beginning to ask tough questions about the economics and patient returns from their computer operations. Is the computer really contributing to faster lab test turnaround? Is the computer really lowering accounts receivables? Do managers really make use of the countless pages of green computer printouts? Not always. As resources become more and more scarce, the tests we apply to continuing support for large computer operations become more rigorous. The result is going to be less, not more, reliance on computers in well-led hospitals.

A large upstate New York tertiary medical center was ahead of its time by not computerizing until the mid 1980s. Although comparably sized New York hospitals were spending millions a year on computer operations, it spent nothing. It refined its manual systems to perfection. The result? They had the lowest accounts receivable status in the state. Their financial statements were always ready by the 10th of the month. Their data keeping systems were limited to information that was really used by management.

While others were busy spending money upgrading their already expensive computers, this hospital spent the money it saved on better wage and benefit programs for its employees and on the latest medical technology. They understood, before the rest of the hospital world, that hospitals can indeed be efficient without computers. Perhaps even more so than with computers.

Planners and marketers

Planners and marketers are the two most popular staff positions. Some hospitals, even some small and medium sized ones, will have planners and marketers by the end of this decade. But many hospitals will close their planning and marketing departments and delegate those responsibilities to senior line managers. As the abilities of hospital leaders increase, there will be less need for dependence on people to tell them how to plan and how to market. Hospital leaders will do it themselves and what they cannot do, they will delegate to specialized consultants rather than operate as in-house staff functions.

Beyond price and service competition

The quality of care in hospitals of the future will increase dramatically due to competitive pressures. Most hospitals are competing with each other based on price and service. Pretty soon the surviving hospitals will improve their services and their prices to the point where the consumers are satisfied. Then what happens? We will begin competing on the basis of patient care quality. Hospitals will compete based on the credentials and quality of physicians and on the outcomes they produce. Medical staffs will come under increased scrutiny by members of the public and by the corporations who purchase health care for their employees.

Companies purchasing services for their employees will demand the best physicians. Hospital leaders will compete for the best to deliver what the purchasers want. Performance data on specific physicians and hospitals will become readily available to the public. It will be data that puts in context the quality of care practiced in our institutions. Infection rates, mortality rates, failed surgeries, and malpractice information will be the subject of further competition just as service and price are today.

When hospitals reach that level, they will truly be competing on quality rather than on service and price. That we are competing at all is good for our consumers. Hospitals are delivering better service and are certainly doing a better job on price than they ever have in the past. Imagine how great it will be for the public when hospitals finally start competing on quality of care. That is going to be the next great challenge for leadership in hospitals.

APPENDIX A

Sample Long-Range Plan Assumptions and Objectives

Assumptions

Patient Acuity—Overall patient acuity is expected to rise as the hospital admits a higher percentage of critically ill patients and as the length of stay decreases as a result of prospective payment system pressures.

Attitude—Physician attitudes toward patients, families and employees need to be enhanced to consistently project a positive image of the Hospital.

Employee Profile—The average age and tenure of employees will rise as lay-offs and schedule reductions cause fewer senior employees to seek employment elsewhere.

HMO/PPO—There will be an increasing emphasis from competitive hospitals and major employers to market HMO and PPO arrangements, representing a threat to our patient-based financial stability.

Hospital and Physician Image—To reduce patient out-migration, hospital and physician community images need to be enhanced, with a particular emphasis on younger (under age 45) individuals and families.

Medicare Reimbursement—Prospective payment systems will remain in effect for Medicare inpatients during the next 36 months and reimbursement per case is expected to decrease.

Objectives

Patient Satisfaction—Implement a statistically significant patient satisfaction measuring program and supporting patient satisfaction programs which achieve a 20 percent increase between 1985 and 1987 in the number of discharged inpatients that give a "highly recommended" rating to Beloit Memorial Hospital.

Ambulatory Surgery Program—Implement a consolidated ambulatory surgery program to meet the outpatient surgery needs of Beloit and surrounding community residents. The ambulatory surgery program will be designed to compete successfully with any outside "surgi-centers" if they are ever set up in the service area of Beloit Memorial Hospital.

Emergency Room—Recruit and retain four emergency residency trained physicians to staff hospital emergency room, establishing the desired level of patient care consistency and high quality care.

Management Development—Implement management development programs to enhance managerial effectiveness and interpersonal skills of all supervisory and management personnel. Separate non-productive management staff and those unable to meet required level of performance as defined by hospital president.

Board Development Plan—In conjunction with evaluation policy, develop and update annually a Board Development

Plan to include educational sessions and periodic board retreats for the purpose of enhancing the overall performance of the board.

Community Perception—Develop community relations program which produces a twenty percent improvement by 1987 in the community preference rating of Beloit Memorial Hospital as measured against baseline data obtained in 1984.

APPENDIX B

Beloit Memorial Hospital, Inc. Policy and Procedure Guide

Subject: Management Evaluation and Compensation Program

Applies To: Vice Presidents, Department Directors and Supervisors

I. Policy

The overall objective of this performance review and compensation program is to retain and reward managers where performance is consistent with organization expectations.

The Management Performance Review Program is designed to enhance strengths and upgrade performance shortcomings in order to improve the performance of individual managers and the overall organization.

Management salary decisions are designed to compensate management for performance while maintaining consistency with the external marketplace.

II. Procedures

A. Performance Evaluation Guidelines

1. *Frequency*

Performance evaluations will be initiated by the personnel department at six (6) months from date of hire or promotion and annually thereafter.

Performance reviews for department directors must be approved by the president. Performance reviews of supervisors must be approved by their respective vice president.

Special evaluations at non-scheduled times are subject to approval by the director of human resources and the president.

2. *Performance Review Format*
Performance reviews will be conducted in a narrative format, using the attached Performance Review Criteria. (Attachment I)

Prior to completing the Performance Review, the individual performing the review will solicit input from the manager being reviewed. This input will include a self-assessment of strengths, areas for improvement, and accomplishments during the review period.

The review meeting itself will be private and permit both parties to fully discuss the review material.

B. Salary Ranges
1. *Revision*
Salary ranges will be reviewed and updated on an annual basis. Ranges will be established to compensate positions consistent with performance and the external marketplace.

2. *Market Surveys*
Salary survey data will be gathered by the director of human resources based on recognized national surveys of hospitals and industry. Sur-

veys are to be used as a general guideline when making salary decisions.

C. Salary Decisions

1. *Salary Increases*

Salary increases are determined based on performance. The president establishes the overall merit management salary increase in January of each year. Managers whose performance is determined to be good to excellent will receive the merit increase. Managers whose performance is less than desired will receive less than the merit increase, and managers whose performance is extremely high may receive more than the merit increase.

2. *Approval and Effective Date*

All salary increases for department directors and vice presidents must be approved by the president. All salary increases for supervisors must be approved by their respective vice president. Increases in pay are effective the beginning of the pay period nearest the date of review.

Any exceptions will be documented in writing and reviewed by the director of human resources and authorized by the president.

Michael E. Rindler
President
June 3, 1986

Management Performance Review Criteria
Beloit Memorial Hospital

Revised: June 3, 1986

The following criteria will be utilized in measuring the performance and effectiveness of the management staff of Beloit Memorial Hospital:

1. Understanding Responsibilities
   A. Maintaining contemporary professional knowledge
   B. Understanding of management expectations
   C. Knowledge of operations of assigned department(s)
   D. Knowledge of outcomes produced by assigned department(s)
2. Initiative
   A. Identifying and implementing operational improvements
   B. Demonstrated problem-solving ability
   C. Ability to constructively express concerns and contrary points of view
3. Responsiveness and Reporting Ability
   A. Ability to work effectively with and enhance performance of supervisor
   B. Ability to respond effectively to supervisory requests
   C. Clarity and organization of written reports
   D. Ability to keep supervisor informed verbally
4. Resource Utilization
   A. Ability to manage man-hours within authorized levels
   B. Effective management of sick time and overtime hours

   C. Ability to manage non-staff expenses within assigned budget

5. Staff Communication
   A. Ability to communicate effectively with subordinate staff
   B. Well-informed about staff issues and problems
   C. Follow-up effectiveness with staff issues
   D. Periodic off-shift presence and staff interaction

6. Results and Objectives
   A. Ability to articulate operating objectives
   B. Accomplishment of assigned objectives

7. Staff Relationships and Development
   A. Ability to critically evaluate subordinates
   B. Ability to set and maintain high operating standards
   C. Achieving excellent staff attitudes and morale
   D. Ability to successfully select and train new employees
   E. Ability to deal effectively with poor performers
   F. Ability to deal effectively with other departments

8. Ability to Delegate
   A. Appropriate selection of delegated tasks
   B. Appropriate use of subordinates to maximize effectiveness

9. Setting a Leadership Example
   A. Promptness and effective use of work time
   B. Demonstrated positive attitude
   C. Observance of hospital policies and regulations
   D. Maintenance of good personal health and professional appearance
   E. Evidence of implemented corporate values in assigned department(s)

10. Attention to Detail
    A. Professional appearance of department(s)
    B. Professional appearance of staff
    C. Attention to operating details of department(s)
11. Summary
    A. Overall description of performance
    B. Areas for improvement

Sample Performance Evaluation: Mr. John Smith, Director of Laboratory Services

June 3, 1986

The following is a performance review for the twelve-month period ending June 3, 1986.

I. Understanding Responsibilities
Mr. Smith has made an effort during this past year to increase his professional knowledge. He has attended one seminar on Laboratory Management and has made an effort to keep current with professional journals. He also visited two other regional laboratories to gain insight about their operations this year. Mr. Smith has an excellent understanding of my expectations, particularly with reference to customer relations and turnaround time for laboratory results. He has an excellent knowledge of the operations within his department and the outcomes produced. His focus on outcomes has been evidenced by implementation of a new series of turnaround time audits and quality assurance audits which are now published monthly.

II. Initiative
Mr. Smith demonstrated initiative during this past year by implementing a patient survey to determine the level of patient satisfaction with laboratory services. This survey included both inpatients and outpatients. Data from the survey helped streamline the admitting process for outpatients. Mr. Smith does need to improve upon his ability to constructively express concerns. He has a tendency to keep the concerns to himself rather than to articulate them.

III. Responsiveness and Reporting Ability
Mr. Smith needs to further understand his responsibility to enhance the effectiveness of his supervisor. There have been several occasions during the past year when opportunities in this regard were missed. Particular reference is made to presentation for a major piece of capital equipment. Mr. Smith responds very promptly to supervisory requests. His written requests are generally well organized; however, capital equipment justifications and staff justifications need to show much improvement. Mr. Smith has a tendency to assume that something is needed just because he requests it. Mr. Smith does keep his supervisor very well informed on both departmental and hospital wide matters.

IV. Resource Utilization
Mr. Smith has done an excellent job in managing his man-hours within authorized levels. He is very aggressive in dealing with employees with sick time problems, and as a consequence has one of the lowest sick time utilizations in the hospital. He also has done an excellent job in managing supply expenses and region expenses for the laboratory.

V. Staff Communication
Mr. Smith does a very good job in communicating with his subordinate staff. He meets weekly with his supervisors and monthly with his general employees. He also makes himself available for ad hoc meetings with both supervisors and employees as the need arises. He has demonstrated an excellent ability to respond to staff issues, and always gets back to staff members with an answer quickly. Mr. Smith has

also demonstrated his interest in off-shift employees by coming in at least once a month for a period of an hour or two on all three shifts.

VI. Results and Objectives

Mr. Smith has demonstrated the ability to articulate excellent operating objectives. This past year, he identified four objectives for his department which were entirely consistent with the corporation's objectives. He further demonstrated his ability to accomplish those objectives.

VII. Staff Relationships and Development

Mr. Smith has demonstrated an ability to critically evaluate his subordinates. He writes excellent performance evaluations and completes them on a timely basis. He has demonstrated the ability to set high operating standards for his departments, particularly in reference to laboratory turnaround test results. He has achieved an excellent level of morale, following the effective dealing with several poor attitude employees who were affecting the morale of the entire department. Mr. Smith has demonstrated his ability to both select and orient new employees. Mr. Smith does need to work on his ability to deal effectively with other departments. During the past year, I received several complaints from his department head peers that he has been uncooperative on cross-departmental matters. Mr. Smith needs to focus less on departmental "turf" and more on positive outcomes for patients.

VIII. Ability to Delegate

Mr. Smith has demonstrated an excellent ability to delegate to his supervisors. He has recently reorganized the supervisory responsibilities to consistently reflect laboratory workload and supervisory capabilities. He uses his subordinates very effectively to maximize his own effectiveness.

IX. Setting a Leadership Example
Mr. Smith sets a good example for leadership in his department. He uses his work time effectively, and sets a good example with reference to work ethic. He has a generally positive attitude, but does tend to hold things in occasionally which negatively affects his personal attitude. He observes all hospital policies and regulations and maintains excellent health and professional appearance. With reference to corporate values, Mr. Smith has taken a personal interest in assuring that each of his employees understands the hospital's five corporate values. He has given specific talks at his monthly meetings as well as shown two films during the past year to strengthen understanding of corporate values.

X. Attention to Detail
Mr. Smith has demonstrated an excellent ability to pay attention to detail. The appearance of his department is excellent, and it is well organized. The appearance of his staff is also excellent, after he dealt with several reluctant employees earlier this past year. He has paid a great deal of attention to the operating details of his departments, particularly as they affect patients. A specific example is the improvement of the turnaround time for laboratory tests in the emergency room so that patients could be discharged quickly.

XI. Summary

Mr. Smith is a very good department director at Beloit Memorial Hospital. He has served in that capacity for five years, and is contributing effectively to the overall success of the hospital.

Mr. Smith has several areas that I would like to see specific improvement on during the next year. These areas are as follows:

1. Ability to constructively express concerns.
2. Improvement of written capital and staff justifications.
3. Improvement on cross-departmental cooperation.

Signed: ______________________________

William Doe
Vice President of Professional Services

____

John Smith
Director of Laboratory Services

APPENDIX C

Position Description: President and Chief Executive Officer

Section 1: Appointment

The board of trustees shall select a president of the corporation. The president shall be the chief executive officer of the corporation, with all of the authority common to the office of the president of a business corporation. The president shall have all authority and responsibility necessary to operate the corporation in all of its activities and departments, subject only to such policies as may be issued by the board of trustees. He or she shall act as the duly authorized representative of the board of trustees and the corporation in all matters in which the board has not formally designated some other person to act.

Section 2: Qualifications

The person appointed as president shall have completed formal education in a graduate program in hospital or business administration in a recognized college or university, and a minimum of seven (7) years experience in a responsible administrative position in a hospital or in the health care field.

Section 3: Accountability

The president shall report to the board of trustees, and as directed to the chairman of the board of trustees between board meetings, and to the executive committee of the board of trustees, at each meeting of those bodies.

Section 4: Compensation

The compensation, terms and conditions of appointment, and services to be rendered to the corporation by the president, shall be established by the board of trustees and updated annually, or more frequently as deemed appropriate by the board of trustees.

Section 5: Authority and Duties

More specifically, the authority and duties of the president shall be:

Board relationships and development

1. Works closely with the board of trustees to enhance its effectiveness in meeting the needs of the corporation.

2. Informs and interests trustees in current trends, issues, problems, activities in health care generally, and community health care needs at the institution to facilitate policy-making.

3. Recommends policy positions concerning legislation, government, and other matters of public policy.

4. Provides comprehensive and accurate information for trustees, for their use in decision-making and policy matters.

5. Assists with identifying potential board members.

6. Submits regularly to the board and its committees, periodic reports showing the professional services and

financial activities of the corporation, and prepares such special reports as may be required by the board.

7. Attends all meetings of the board and its committees.

8. Interprets the meaning of these by-laws and all other regulations and policies adopted by the board as they may apply in case of uncertainty or dispute, to have the meaning that the president has been authorized and empowered by the board to be the chief executive officer of the corporation, and the decision of the president shall govern, unless otherwise specifically overruled by the actions of the board of trustees.

Planning

1. Participates with the board in charting the course of the corporation in response to the needs of the community.

2. Evaluates the effects of external forces on the corporation and integrates appropriate responses into the corporation's short and long-range plans.

3. Recommends long-range plans to the board which support the corporation's Statement of Mission and Statement of Corporate Goals.

4. Completes an annual operating plan to facilitate achievement of goals established in the corporation's long-range plan.

Management and professional staff

1. Ensures the attainment of corporation goals through the selection, development, motivation, and evaluation of all corporate management and professional staff.

2. Develops and implements plan of organization to meet the needs of the corporation.

3. Selects, employs, controls, and discharges all management and professional staff members of the corporation.

4. Establishes formal responsibilities and accountabilities of all members of the management and professional staff and evaluates their performance regularly.

5. Establishes compensation and benefits for all members of the management and professional staff.

6. Negotiates professional contracts and ensures that appropriate salary or contractual rates are developed and maintained.

Human resource management

1. Ensures that patient care and operational needs of the corporation are attained through the selection, training, motivation and evaluation of all employees of the corporation.

2. Implements appropriate staffing levels and a plan of departmentalization to facilitate effective delivery of patient care and support services.

3. Specifies personnel accountability and ensures that performance is evaluated regularly.

4. Establishes compensation and benefits consistent with board-approved limitations.

Quality of health care services

1. Monitors the adequacy of the corporation's medical activities, appointments, reappointments and medical

staff privileges the policies needed to assure quality health care services, through coordination with the board, medical staff, and patient care staff.

2. Creates an operating environment which facilitates the effective practice of medicine by the physician members of the medical staff.

3. Consults with leaders of the medical and dental staff concerning patient care needs and allocation of resources to effectively meet those needs.

4. Represents the board of trustees before the medical staff of Beloit Memorial Hospital.

5. Coordinates the recruitment and retention of members of the medical staff of Beloit Memorial Hospital.

Allocation of resources

1. Promotes delivery of health care services in a cost effective manner consistent with maintenance of an acceptable level of quality.

2. Assures the sound fiscal operation of the corporation, including developing a comprehensive annual operating budget and implementing that budget following board approval.

3. Develops a capital equipment budget and implements that budget following board approval.

4. Plans the use and maintenance of the physical resources of the corporation.

5. Insures all corporation property against damage.

6. Supervises all business affairs of the corporation and

ensures that all funds are collected and expended to maximize the operating effectiveness of the corporation.

7. Arranges contractual relationships with consultants, contractors, architects, and similar professionals in planning and developing facilities, finances and personnel programs.

8. Signs contracts or other instruments as the authorized representative of the corporation, except in cases where execution shall have been expressly delegated by law, or the board of trustees, to somc other officer or agent of the corporation.

Compliance with regulations

1. Ensures compliance with regulations governing the corporation and the rules of accrediting bodies by continually monitoring the corporation's activities and initiating changes as required.

2. Participation in litigation against the corporation.

3. Recommends to the board of trustees the need to institute litigation.

4. Approves final settlements of all lawsuits against the corporation.

Promotion of the corporation

1. Encourages the integration of the corporation with the community by implementing effective communication and community relations programs.

2. Represents the board of trustees to the community.

3. Initiates, develops, and maintains cooperative rela-

tionships with the business community and other regional health care providers.

4. Generates community involvement through auxiliary, volunteer and staff programs.

5. Speaks before community and business groups about health care problems and the corporation's programs to meet community health care needs.

General

1. Provides overall leadership and coordinates activities of all aspects of the corporation, with the objective that the entire corporation will function as an effective unit, providing the highest quality patient care and support services consistent with available resources.

2. Maintains contemporary knowledge on ideas and developments in all phases of hospital administration to the end that the president shall provide leadership for all personnel of the corporation, the board of trustees, and the medical staff.

3. Promulgates and enforces all rules and regulations for the proper conduct of the corporation and its purposes made by and under the authority of the board of trustees. Formulates, establishes, and enforces such additional procedures, rules and regulations as may be necessary to provide for the proper admission, care, safety, and discharge of patients.

APPPENDIX D

Chief Executive Office Performance Evaluation Policy

I. Purpose

It is the policy of XYZ Hospital, Inc. to utilize a formal performance evaluation program for the president and chief executive officer. The purpose of this program is to maximize the effectiveness of the president and to promote an effective working relationship between the board of trustees and the corporation president. Additionally, the program is intended to enhance the professional development of the president so that he can maximize his contribution to the organization.

II. Performance evaluation period

The evaluation period shall be twelve months, commencing on January 1 of each year. The formal annual performance review shall take place in February of each year. The mid-year informal evaluation shall take place in July of each year.

III. Performance evaluation committee

A chief executive officer evaluation committee shall be established to perform the duties as defined in this policy. The committee shall consist of the chairman of the board and two other trustees to be selected by the chairman.

The committee shall meet as often as necessary. At a minimum, the committee shall meet at the beginning of the evaluation period to establish, in conjunction with the board and the president, mutually agreed upon performance goals for the evaluation period. Additionally, the committee shall meet in the middle of the evaluation period to informally apprise the president of his performance, and at the end of the evaluation period to administer the formal performance evaluation.

IV. Performance evaluation criteria

There shall be three overall criteria on which the performance evaluation is based. These are:

A. *Performance goals*

Three to four overall goals which are mutually agreed upon by the evaluation committee, the board, and the president. These areas shall be broad in scope but have definitive and measurable outcomes.

B. *Position responsibilities*

Assessment of the president's overall performance on the position responsibilities as defined in Article ABC of the by-laws of the corporation.

C. *Summary*

A summary section which rates the overall performance of the president. This summary section shall include an identification of significant accomplishments during the evaluation period and the identification of areas which need further development by the president.

V. Evaluation procedure

The procedure to be used in evaluating the performance of the president is as follows:

A. *Goal establishment*

In October, the president shall draft approximately four overall performance goals for the upcoming evaluation period. The goals shall be definitive in nature and shall be the overall priorities of the president during the evaluation period. These goals will be reviewed and approved by the performance evaluation committee and recommended to the full board for approval by December.

B. *Informal review*

The performance evaluation committee shall meet informally with the president in July to provide informal feedback. Additionally, the chairman shall regularly provide the president with informal feedback concerning his performance.

C. *Formal performance evaluation*

The formal performance evaluation shall be at the end of the evaluation period. Preceding the evaluation meeting, the president shall prepare for the performance evaluation committee a summary of progress on the performance goals and a summary of the significant accomplishments during the evaluation period. Also preceding the performance review meeting, the chairman shall provide the president with a copy of the written performance evaluation for review and comment.

The performance evaluation committee shall meet personally with the president to discuss the formal performance review. This review shall include evaluation of accomplishment of performance goals, performance on job responsibilities, and a summary of overall performance.

D. *Report to the board of trustees*
The chairman will provide an oral report to the full board of trustees at the next regular board meeting following the performance evaluation session.

VI. Compensation and benefits
The performance evaluation committee is responsible for establishing the salary and fringe benefit program for the president. The overall purpose of the compensation and benefit program shall be to maximize motivation and performance of the president. Additionally, the compensation and benefit program shall be structured to encourage the retention of a qualified president who is meeting the expectations of the board of trustees.

The performance evaluation committee shall consult whatever sources it deems necessary to establish the compensation and benefit program for the chief executive officer. An evaluation of the president's compensation and benefit program shall take place at least annually, or more frequently as determined by the performance evaluation committee.

VII. Policy review

This policy shall be reviewed annually by the performance evaluation committee and recommendations for changes, as necessary, shall be submitted by the chairman to the full board of trustees for approval.

REFERENCES

1 1986 Directory: American Association of Healthcare Consultants.

2 Peters, Thomas J., and Waterman Jr., Robert H., *In Search of Excellence* (New York: Harper and Row Publishers, 1980), p. 13.

3 Hayes, Robert H., and Abernathy, William J., ''Managing Our Way to Economic Decline,'' *Harvard Business Review,* (July-August, 1980), pp. 70-71.

4 Albrecht, Karl, and Zemke, Ron, *Service America* (Homewood, Illinois: Dow Jones-Irwin, 1985), pp. 104-105.

5 Ibid., pp. 144-145.

6 Ibid.

7 Ibid., p. 6.

8 Ibid., p. 27.

9 Ibid., p. 124.

10 Peters, Thomas J., and Waterman Jr., Robert H., p. 312.

11 Umdenstock, Richard J., and Hageman, Winifred, *Hospital Corporate Leadership* (Chicago: American Hospital Publishing, Inc., 1984), pp. 9-10.

Index